Colloidal Silver

Medical Uses, Toxicology and Manufacture

Third Edition   **By John W Hill**

ISBN-13: 978-1-884979-08-8
ISBN-10: 1-884979-08-4

Library of Congress Control No.: 2009902408

BISAC Subject Headings:

MED004000	**MEDICAL** / Alternative Medicine	
MED023000	**MEDICAL** / Drug Guides	
MED039000	**MEDICAL** / History	
MED040000	**MEDICAL** / Holistic Medicine	
MED022090	**MEDICAL** / Infectious Diseases	
MED072000	**MEDICAL** / Pharmacy	
HEA032000	**HEALTH & FITNESS** / Alternative Therapies	
HEA011000	**HEALTH & FITNESS** / Herbal Medications	

Published by: Clear Springs Press, LLC

http://www.clspress.com/contact.html

Where to Order this Book

(1) You can order online from Amazon at:

http://www.amazon.com

Search for this book by title or by the ISBN number:

ISBN-13: 978-1-884979-08-8
ISBN-10: 1-884979-08-4

(2) For wholesale and bulk orders contact:

> Clear Springs Press
> http://www.clspress.com/contact.html

(3) You may also place wholesale or bookstore orders with Ingram Book Group

http://www.ingrampublisherservices.com/retailer/default.asp

One Ingram Blvd.
P.O. Box 3006
LaVergne, TN 37086-1986

(866) 400-5351

Retailer@ingrampublisherservices.com

_____

For all other inquiries, contact the publisher by logging onto the website and using the contact form.

Published by: Clear Springs Press, LLC

http://www.clspress.com/contact.html

Contents

Terminology

Here are some common terms used in discussing colloidal silver and silver products:

Ag - The symbol for silver.

Ag$^+$ - The symbol for a silver ion.

Agglomeration - Agglomeration is the process whereby smaller particles combine to form larger particles. Unstable silver colloids may undergo agglomeration that results in the precipitation of silver particles out of suspension.

Argyria - A condition caused by ingesting too much silver, ingesting it too quickly, or ingesting more toxic forms of silver. This condition is characterized by silver deposition in the skin and other body tissues. The characteristic symptom is the skin turning blue or grey.

Bacteriostatic - Capable of inhibiting the growth of a microorganism.

Bactericidal - Capable of killing a microorganism.

Colloid - A chemical mixture where one substance is dispersed evenly throughout another. The particles of the dispersed substance are only suspended in the mixture, unlike a solution, where they are completely dissolved within. This occurs because the particles in a colloid are small enough to be dispersed evenly and maintain a homogenous appearance, but large enough to scatter light and not dissolve.

Colloidal Silver – By definition, colloidal silver is a suspension of silver particles in water. The term is frequently used, however, to describe a variety of medicinal or nutritional products, some of which may not be true colloids.

Hemolysis - The destruction of red blood cells.

In vitro - In a test tube or a petri dish, not a live body.

In vivo - In a real life situation, in a live body.

Ion – An ion is an atom which has lost or gained one or more electrons and is left with a positive or negative charge.

Leukocyte - White blood cells.

Luekocytosis - An elevation in leukocyte count.

Leukopenia - A decrease in leukocyte count.

MIC - Minimum inhibitory concentration. The lowest level at which the reproduction of a microorganism is stopped.

PPM - Parts per million of a solution, suspension, or mixture. With colloidal silver, 1PPM is the equivalent of 1 milligram of silver in a liter of water.

Osteomyelitis - Bone infection.

Oligodynamic - Effective in small quantities.

Sepsis - Infection in the blood stream.

Solution - A homogeneous mixture composed of two or more substances. In a solution, a solute is dissolved in a solvent. An example is silver nitrate dissolved in water.

Suspension - A heterogeneous fluid containing solid particles that are sufficiently large for sedimentation, generally larger than one micron. Unlike colloids, suspensions will eventually settle.

Tyndall Effect - The effect of light scattering by colloidal or suspended particles. A light beam passing through a colloidal suspension in a liquid casts a visible beam.

Preface

Colloidal Silver in various forms was used as a mainstream medicine in the late 1800's and early 1900's. It was replaced by modern antibiotics in the mid 1900's and rediscovered in the 1980's and 1990's. As an unapproved new drug or a nutritional supplement, depending on the language used to describe it, it was an orphan looking for a home. It did, however, attract a lot of attention. After significant research and development by scientists and inventors, new products, production methods, and applications are appearing. There has recently been a number of new patents issued and applied for regarding colloidal silver, silver products and their medical applications. In recent years, there have also been hundreds of new articles published in scientific and medical journals that relate to silver, colloidal silver, and nano-silver in some fashion.

Silver, silver colloids, and silver salts have a long history of use in medicine as antiseptics and antibiotics. Some forms of colloidal silver are so easy to make that anyone can make them in their kitchen. The potential of having a super antibiotic that anyone can make for pennies in their kitchen has caught the interest of many individuals.

Colloidal Silver is not approved by the FDA. It is, however, widely sold as a nutritional supplement. When it is sold as a nutritional supplement, colloidal silver manufacturers are banned from providing consumers any information about its safe and effective usage.

This document is a review of medical and scientific literature related to colloidal silver. This book is not intended to be construed as medical advice. If you have a medical condition that you intend to treat with colloidal silver, please find an open-minded physician to assist you in the proper diagnosis and care of your condition.

With the information in this book you can manufacture colloidal silver for pennies per gallon rather than have to purchase it for dollars per ounce. This makes it especially important to resist the temptation to over use or misuse it.

Brief History of Silver and Silver Colloids in Medicine

Silver has been used as a medicine and preservative by many cultures throughout history. The Greeks, Romans, Egyptians, and others used silver vessels for water and other liquids to keep them fresh. Pioneers trekking across the Wild West generations ago faced many hardships. Keeping safe drinking water was one of them. Bacteria, algae, etc. found a fertile breeding ground in the wooden water casks that were carried on the wagons. They placed silver and copper coins in the casks to retard the growth of these spoilage organisms. They also put silver dollars in their milk to keep it fresh.

Silver water purification filters and tablets manufactured in Switzerland are used by many nations and international airlines. Silver is also used in the water purification systems of space craft. Preventing the growth of algae and bacteria in swimming pools is another problem that people face today. Electrical ionization units that impregnate the water with silver and copper ions are available today that sanitize the pool water without the harsh effects of chlorine.

Medical applications of silver were recognized by the ancient Egyptians, Greeks, Romans, and in the alchemical writings of Paracelsus. Following the discovery of bacteria as a cause of disease, several physicians discovered the antibacterial qualities of silver and applied them to their practice of medicine. They used silver nitrate successfully in the treatment of skin ulcers, compound fractures, and suppurating wounds.

In 1881, Carl Crede pioneered the installation of 2% silver nitrate in the eye of neonates to prevent gonorrheal ophthalmia, a technique which has been in widespread use ever since. Von Naegeli and others in 1893 realized that the antibacterial effects of silver were primarily due to the silver ion. He coined the term oligodynamic to mean that a small amount of silver is released from the metallic surface when placed in contact with liquids.

In the early 1900's silver foil dressings were used for wounds. These dressings were used extensively until just after World War II, and were listed in the Physician's Desk Reference until 1955.

In the early 1970's, Drs. Becker, Marino, and Spadaro, of the Veterans Administration Hospital in Syracuse, New York, pioneered the study of implanted silver wires and electrodes and silver-coated fabrics for the treatment of complex bone infections.

Dr. A. B. Flick developed broader clinical applications for silver nylon fabrics, first in partnership with Dr. Becker and later independently. Other university centered research teams also investigated the wound healing properties of silver plated fabrics applied with the application of an electrical potential. The result was the commercial introduction of silver dressings for wound healing and burns.

Silver sulfadiazine ointment is the number one treatment for burns in U.S. burn centers. Silver coated catheters and silver heart valves are used because they stop the bacterial growth that was commonplace with the old ones. To protect us from food poisoning, silver particles are now being put in cutting boards, table tops, surface disinfectants, washing machines, and refrigerators. Silver is now being used in clothing, for the military, sportsman and businessman. It is woven and impregnated into the fabric to kill bacteria that cause body odor and clothing odors.

In contemporary times, colloidal silver as a medicinal substance for internal use is something of an orphan. It is popular among alternative medicine enthusiasts but is not approved by the FDA.

Silver was used as a medicine in the late 1800's and early 1900's. While several metal salts and compounds demonstrated strong germicidal properties, silver alone showed both strong germicidal properties and low or no toxicity to humans. The colloidal state proved to be the most effective form because it lacked the caustic properties of salts (such as silver nitrate) and demonstrated a high level of activity with very low concentrations.

Medicinal silver compounds were in widespread use in the late 1800's and early 1900's. By 1940, there were approximately four dozen different silver compounds on the market being used to treat every known infectious disease.

These different silver preparations were drastically different from each other. Some were true colloids of silver, others were silver salts or other compounds of silver. Many were silver proteinates. The actual silver content also varied widely, with some products containing as much as 30% silver by weight.

With the discovery of antibiotics, interest in silver, as an anti-microbial medicine, declined. There were, at that time, no antibiotic resistant strains of disease organisms and there was a lot of excitement over the new wonder drugs.

In Ayurvedic medicine silver is used in small amounts as a tonic or elixir or rejuvenative agent for patients debilitated by age or disease. Silver was also used in homeopathic medicine. The dilute concentrations were in the same range as the modern low concentrations of colloidal silver.

Recently, with the development of antibiotic resistance in many diseases and the increase in new strains of bacteria and viruses worldwide, there is renewed interest in silver. Large companies are developing and introducing new silver compounds for a variety of anti-microbial applications, including protection against the spread of the AIDS virus. (2)

Today, colloidal silver is sold as a trace mineral supplement without medical claims or claims of specific benefits. Its need, or lack thereof, in human nutrition is not scientifically established. It remains popular as an "alternative" health care modality because of the large number of anecdotal reports of positive benefits.

The Different Forms of Colloidal Silver

A colloid is a very small particle which remains suspended in water without actually forming an ionic solution. A colloid of silver is a very small particle of metallic silver suspended in water. The atomic micro-clusters of silver atoms found in colloidal silver range in size between approximately 0.001 and 0.01 microns. The small size means a very large surface area of silver per unit volume of silver. This small size, with its large surface area to volume ratio, enhances the surface chemistry of silver and dramatically increases the reactivity of silver with the substances that it comes in contact with. These particles are smaller than the individual cells of bacteria and some of the particles are smaller even than viruses.

An "ionic" silver compound, by contrast, is one which will dissolve in water. Being soluble, its chemical reactivity is even higher than that of a colloidal suspension. Ionic silver compounds, or silver salts, are, however, more toxic to living systems than colloidal suspensions. Silver Nitrate has been used as a germicide and even as an internal medicine in the past. As a germicide, it is extremely effective but can be caustic and irritating to tissues and only a fool would swallow the stuff. Other ionic compounds have varying degrees of effectiveness as a germicide and varying degrees of toxicity as well.

Many of the colloidal silver products on the market are a blend of ionic silver and suspensions of pure metallic silver in water. Some manufacturers bind the silver to a protein or polymer molecule to stabilize it and prevent precipitation. There is some debate about which form is best.

Here are some of the major types of silver products that are or have been produced and used:

Electro-colloidal Silver – This type of silver is produced by an electrolytic process or some version of electric arc. The concentration is typically from 1 to 20 PPM for the low voltage cathodic process.

Mild silver Protein (MSP): Silver colloids are precipitated from a silver salt by a reducing agent and chemically bonded to a protein. The concentration may vary from 20 PPM to 5,000 PPM.

Powdered Silver: A very high voltage is used to disintegrate the silver. This process could be described as both a thermal and electrical process.

Ground Silver: In this process, silver was ground to a fine powder. This process was abandoned because the silver particles were too large.

Silver salts: These are ionic silver compounds that are produced chemically.

There are a number of silver compounds that have been used in medicine or are being used now. These include silver sulfadiazine, silver nitrate, silver citrate, silver iodide, silver chloride, silver lactate, silver oxide and silver picrate.

In the past, several colloidal silver products were listed in the United States Pharmacopoeia (U.S.P.) and the National Formulary (N.F.). (64) These included colloidal silver iodide containing 18-22 percent silver (diluted to 0.05-10 percent silver for local use) and strong silver protein containing 7.5-8.5 percent silver (diluted to 0.5-10 percent). None of these formerly recognized colloidal silver preparations have been official in the U.S.P. or the N.F. since 1975. (64)

Colloidal Silver websites on the internet often present contradictory opinions on the virtues of different types of silver products. Some claim that ionic silver is more effective while others claim that colloidal silver is more effective. Still others claim that mild silver protein or compounds like silver citrate are superior.

An ion is an atom which has lost or gained one or more electrons and is left with a positive or negative charge. While metallic silver is regarded to be insoluble in water, it is known that a small amount is dispersed in the water. It is unclear exactly what form this dispersal is in.

14

One theory is that a small amount of silver goes into solution by forming a compound of AgOH with the free hydroxyl radicals in the water. Another is that silver reacts with dissolved carbon dioxide to produce a compound of Ag_2CO_3. Either of these compounds could produce a low concentration of silver ions in solution.

In the debate over colloidal versus ionic silver, it appears that some producers regard electrically charged microclusters of metallic silver to be ions. In addition to the differences in the definition of ionic, there is some challenge in measuring the relative composition of ions versus colloidal particles in particular products.

Absorption and Elimination of Silver

Two very important factors in the safety of silver products are the total accumulated dose of silver and how quickly it was consumed. The rate of consumption is probably more important than the total quantity because there is an excretion process. If the intake exceeds the body's ability to eliminate the silver, it accumulates in the tissues. An estimation of the body's ability to eliminate silver is then critical to understanding what dosage is toxic.

It appears that colloidal silver is absorbed orally through the GI tract, through the nasal mucosa, sublingually, and rectally. Some individuals also have reported injecting colloidal silver or administering it intravenously.

None of the old medical literature that I was able to find gave a satisfactory assessment of the absorption, retention, and excretion of colloidal silver. The old literature suggested that silver is eliminated primarily through the feces with active biliary excretion. Even inhaled silver is eliminated through the feces. (63)

One individual, Roger Altman, Eng.Sc.D., conducted independent research without support or funding to find some of the answers to these questions. He made careful measurements of the silver that he consumed and the silver that he excreted in urine, feces, hair, nails, sweat, etc. From his carefully collected data, we now have an indication of how these processes work.

Dr. Altman consumed 2.34 mg of silver daily for several months then measured the total silver excreted from his body over a 24 hour period. He concluded that silver is excreted easily from the body, primarily in the urine. The total silver excreted during this particular measurement period exceeded the amount consumed during that period. This is accounted for by the variability of the amount of waste (urine, feces, etc.) eliminated from the body and the amount of silver consumed through food and water, etc. It does point out that silver is eliminated from the body much more efficiently than we previously thought. It may also explain why there have been very few cases of argyria reported by individuals using low dosage electrocolloidal silver. The colloidal silver that he was using was electrocolloidal silver made by the high voltage DC (180 VDC) process. (74)

This is only one set of measurements on one individual. However, the data is carefully obtained by a scientifically trained individual using modern analytical tools. It suggests that a healthy adult can consume approximately 2 mg of colloidal silver per day without risk. This data is insufficient, however, to assume that the same situation will prevail in other individuals. Someone with kidney disease, for example, may have difficulty eliminating silver and may risk toxicity with prophylactic consumption.

The following quotations are taken from the conclusion of the 24 hour silver balance test (daily intake=2.34 mg):

1. "Silver is excreted easily from the body, primarily in the urine."

2. "More silver was measured leaving the body than entering during a 24hour period. This probably can be accounted for by the variability of the total amount of urine and feces produced on a day to day basis, i.e., body tissue acts as a "flywheel" retaining and excreting more or less silver depending on the daily volume of bodily waste generated." [Author's note: There is also silver intake from food and water that would need to be accounted for].

3. "Since the same daily amount of silver had been taken for several months prior to this 24 hour test, it is reasonable to conclude that the total amount of silver residing in the body tissue is many times that of the daily amount eliminated (this conclusion is supported by additional evidence given later). Therefore, it seems quite possible that CS taken prophylacticly offers better protection than CS taken only at the onset of illness."

[Author's note: The raw data suggests that very little silver goes into hair, nails, or perspiration.]

Dr. Altman also ran a measurement of silver elimination for 100 days following the cessation of silver intake. The elimination is primarily through the urine the first five days after ceasing silver intake. This phase is followed by a period of increased elimination of silver from the tissues. The later phase appears to be dominated by elimination of silver through the feces. Elimination through the feces is the major excretion pathway from day 33 to 96. He also noted that the intake of extra water increased the elimination of silver in the urine in almost direct proportion to the increase in water intake.

Dr. Altman's conclusions are:

"Ingestion of properly prepared CS does not result in silver accumulating in the body."

"There is no evidence that silver deposits significantly in hair or fingernails and, in fact, the data support the conclusion that after taking more than 2 mg of CS per day for several months, silver seems to be purged from the body (mostly through urine) at about the same rate at which it is consumed."

"Furthermore, upon terminating CS intake, it appears that as much as half of the silver residing in body tissue will be purged through urine and feces, but more and more through feces as time goes on, in less than a month. Even this relatively short residence time could be reduced substantially if several liters of water were consumed daily."

Another report on silver, the EPA IRIS Report (Integrated Risk Information Systems), states that a number of tests were completed to test the absorption and retention of ingested silver in a number of animals, including primates. In its conclusion, the test work indicated that between 90-99% of ingested silver was excreted on the second day after ingestion, and greater than 99% was excreted in less than a week. So, in other words, almost all of the ingested silver was out of the body in only two days, and most of the rest was out of the body in a week. (103)

The available information suggests that silver salts are clearly more toxic than silver proteins or colloidal silver. It is possible to produce a variety of silver salts and other silver compounds in some manufacturing processes. These may be left over from the materials used in the manufacturing process or may be produced by the manufacturing process as a by product, especially if impure materials are used. Some methods of producing silver colloids chemically use silver nitrate as one of the ingredients and there may be traces of it remaining in the mixture.

For someone using colloidal silver, it is important to estimate the total number of milligrams of silver in a dose and the total number of milligrams consumed over the course of treatment.

Here is a summary of reference points to work from:

- One tsp contains 5 ml of liquid.

- One PPM concentration is the same as 1 milligram (mg) per liter.

- (Example: 10 PPM colloidal silver contains 10 mg of silver in one liter of liquid.)

- (Example: One tsp of 10 PPM colloidal silver contains 50 micrograms of silver.)

- The EPA reference dose for a 160 pound adult (the average amount consumed per day in food and water) is 364 micrograms per day.

- The EPA critical dose for a 160 pound adult (the amount that should not be exceeded in daily consumption) is 1.09 milligrams per day.

- The EPA proposed limit for silver in drinking water is: 0.1 mg per liter (0.1 PPM).

- The average person consumes approximately 90 mcg of silver per day in their food.

- References (8) and (70) suggest that the estimated total dosage of mild silver protein required to treat serious infections such as LYME disease is: Approximately 18 to 90 milligrams of silver over the period of one month.

- The estimated accumulated dosage required to produce argyria is approximately one to six grams of silver, depending on the reference cited. Some references state as high as 50 grams. (1)(62)

- The estimated single dose lethal quantity of silver is approximately ten grams of silver. (Note: This estimate is for silver nitrate which is much more toxic than colloidal silver.) (56)

While colloidal silver has been injected intramuscularly and intravenously, the most common method of administration is orally. Li and Zhu (136) have demonstrated that that nanoparticle silver reacts readily with hydrochloric acid. This is in contrast to the fact that metallic silver does not react readily with hydrochloric acid. We can, therefore, assume that the colloidal silver that is swallowed is converted to silver chloride by the hydrochloric acid in the stomach. When the stomach contents are emptied into the intestines, they are combined with bicarbonate which neutralizes the stomach acid and converts the medium from acid to alkaline. This would cause the silver chloride to precipitate, probably into a colloidal form.

It has not been clearly established how much colloidal silver enters the blood as silver particles and how much has been converted into chloride or protein bound forms.

Silver Toxicity - How much is Harmful?

Can Colloidal Silver harm you? Almost anything can be harmful if used in excess. This includes commonly used drugs and even common foods. Potatoes, tomatoes, wheat, mushrooms, and many other common foods contain toxins and/or carcinogens or even mostly harmless substances which can be harmful to susceptible individuals. They don't usually harm us because we limit their consumption to levels that our body can adapt to, and metabolize.

The bottom line is that small doses of silver seem harmless for most people while large doses taken in great excess can be toxic. So the question is: What constitutes a small safe amount and what constitutes a large potentially harmful amount?

Unfortunately, there is no definitive answer to that question. There is, however, some information available that can serve as points of reference from which an "estimate" can be made.

Much of the toxicological data is derived from data on silver salts and silver proteins with much higher silver content than current electrocolloidal products. It is also true that colloidal silver, silver salts, and silver proteins cannot be assumed to produce the same results or have the same toxicities.

In addition to argyria, the intake of very large doses (far in excess of the amount that causes discoloration of the skin) of silver can cause neurological damage, organ damage, and arteriosclerosis.

In one research project, dogs died from injections of a type of protein bound silver in dosages ranging from 500 mg to 1.9 grams of silver depending on the dosage and frequency of administration. (46) This was equivalent in silver content to giving a 150 pound adult between 150 and 570 liters of 10 PPM colloidal silver, or between 75 and 285 liters of 20 PPM colloidal silver, or between 50 and 190 liters of 30 PPM colloidal silver. The 10 gram estimated lethal dose for humans from Goodman and Gillman (56) is equivalent in silver content to 1000 liters of 10 PPM colloidal silver.

In this study (46), the authors were attempting to cause anemia in dogs for experimental purposes rather than test the effect or safety of colloidal silver. They injected Collargol, which contains approximately 87% silver with the remainder being albuminous proteins.

In one test, they injected 500 mg of Collargol into a 23 kg dog. The dog died 12 hours later. They further noted that doses of 1.3 to 1.5 grams of Collargol are tolerated (before death occurs) if divided and given at the proper intervals over a period of 3 to 7 days. Single doses of 200 to 300 mg were well tolerated. Death usually followed a single large dose.

Upon necropsy, the following pathological changes were noted:

(1) There was moderate congestion and marked edema of the lungs.

(2) The reticuloendothelial cells of the liver and spleen contained coarse silver deposits. So did lymph nodes, bone marrow, and to a lesser degree, the kidneys.

(3) The bone marrow showed slight to marked hyperplasia with no death to the parent cells and contained many mononuclear cells filled with brown (silver) pigment.

(4) The hematocrit dropped 10 to 14 percent.

(5) There was a slimy exudate from the nose.

(6) Those overdosed over a longer time period became emaciated.

The administration of smaller doses, 20 to 50 mg over intervals resulted in mild leukocytosis and an increase in hematocrit.

The authors reference another article in which a human died two hours after receiving an intravenous injection of 50 mg Collargol. An autopsy revealed changes nearly identical to those described for the dogs.

More recently, Motohashi performed an experiment in which Collargum was injected into rabbits. After the injection, he observed that the hemophages began "ingesting the animal's own erythrocytes abnormally." He determined that the minimum dose of injected Collargum into rabbits which caused increased hemophage activity was 1 cc of a 1:10000 dillution per kilogram of weight. (123)

In another case (47), an individual ingested an estimated 124 grams of silver nitrate over a period of 9 years. She developed argyria and an assortment of neurological symptoms as well. The authors note that the silver tended to complex with sulfur in the form of Ag_2S. A moderate presence of silver-sulfur granules were seen in the perineural tissue, in the peripheral nerves and along the elastic fibers, and to a lesser extent along the collagenous fibers, and in macrophages. These deposits were noted to have an affinity for basal membranes. The neurological manifestations included taste and smell disorders, vertigo, and hyeresthesia. This report is often used by critics to attribute neurological disorders to colloidal silver consumption. For comparisons to be meaningful, differences in dosage regimens must be accounted for.

It may be helpful to put this in perspective with the quantity of silver that is consumed in food and drinking water from natural sources. The EPA publishes a reference dose (RFD) for silver which is an estimate of daily exposure to the entire population that is unlikely to be associated with a significant risk of adverse effects over a lifetime. The current RFD for oral silver exposure is 5 micrograms/kg/day with a critical dose estimated at 14 micrograms/kg/day. The maximum contaminant level proposed by the EPA for silver in the drinking water is less than 0.1 mg/L (less than 0.1 PPM).

Based on this RFD, a 150 pound adult should not exceed 350 micrograms/day. If the silver in drinking water meets EPA standards, an average person drinking 2 liters per day will consume less than 200 micrograms of silver. In addition the daily diet may contain about 90 micrograms of silver. (63) 350 micrograms of silver is equivalent to 70 milliliters (14 tsp) of 5 PPM colloidal silver. This is the amount that the EPA standards permit an individual to consume from natural sources.

Some researchers have suggested that a deficiency of selenium and vitamin E may increase the susceptibility to systemic silver toxicity. It was hypothesized that silver toxicity, as manifested by liver necrosis in laboratory rats, was due to silver induced inhibition of the synthesis of the seleno-enzyme glutathione peroxidase. Bunyan, et. al., showed that rats supplemented with selenium or vitamin E tolerated a silver exposure of as high as 140 mcg/kg/day. (63)

It is also necessary to remember that some individuals have allergies to specific metals. Nickel, copper, silver, and other metals have been known to cause allergic reactions. Be certain that you are not allergic to silver before taking colloidal silver.

Silver Toxicity Summary

It appears that healthy adults may be able to take as much as 2 mg of colloidal silver per day without overwhelming the body's elimination mechanisms. Additional research needs to be done to test this hypothesis.

Individuals with kidney disease may be at increased risk for developing silver toxicity. This is a reasonable assumption since it appears that the kidneys are a major pathway in eliminating silver from the body. Drinking extra water increases silver elimination and may reduce silver accumulation and risk of toxicity.

Liver disease may increase silver toxicity. Silver may interfere with certain metaloenzymes in the liver, especially if there is a deficiency of selenium or vitamin E. Taking extra supplements of selenium and vitamin E may reduce an individual's susceptibility to silver toxicity. This is based on the finding that supplementation decreased liver toxicity in rats and that rats deficient in these nutrients were more susceptible to silver toxicity.

Some silver salts are significantly more toxic than colloidal silver, and silver compounds introduce many additional variables.

Larger doses and more concentrated forms of silver increase risk of toxicity and argyria since they may exceed the body's ability to eliminate the excess silver.

Risk of silver toxicity or argyria may be reduced by avoiding any silver consumption for a period of three to four months after the completion of a therapeutic regimen. Based on Dr. Altman's experiment, this would give the body time to eliminate much of the stored silver in the body before continuing treatment.

The risk of silver toxicity and argyria may be reduced if the total cumulative dosage is kept under one gram of silver, especially if large doses are being consumed or there is kidney or liver dysfunction present.

Argyria

Most of the medical literature states that the only adverse effect of excess consumption of silver or silver products is a condition called argyria. Argyria is characterized by gray to gray-black staining of the skin and mucous membranes produced by silver deposition. This coloration is permanent. Most authorities state that argyria is disfiguring because of the discoloration of the skin but has no other harmful consequences. Hill and Pillsbury note in their 1939 book Argyria, "A striking feature of argyria is the absence of any evidence that the deposits of silver produce any significant physiologic disturbance of the involved organs or tissue.... Aside from the pigment deposit, the gross and microscopic appearance of the involved tissues is normal. Argyria is, therefore, of significance only from the standpoint of cosmetic appearance." (1)

Hill and Pillsbury could only find 239 reported cases of argyria by 1939. At this time, silver had been in widespread use for over four decades. Most of the cases involved chronic use ranging from 3 to 25 years. Over half of the cases were associated with silver nitrate usage. Even so, they concluded that even with silver nitrate "the danger of argyria is very slight if the total amount injested by mouth is below six grams." (1)

It is estimated that, in recent years, many thousands of individuals have consumed colloidal silver products with no adverse effects or indications of argyria. There have been, however, a very small number of cases and they have achieved notoriety.

One well publicized example is the case of Rosemary Jacobs. Rosemary's case was reported in The New England Journal of Medicine, Volume 340:1554 May 20, 1999 Number 20. The journal states, "A 56-year-old woman has had discolored skin since the age of 14. At the age of 11, the patient was given nose drops of unknown composition for 'allergies' and three years later her skin turned gray." Silver nitrate nose drops were commonly prescribed in that era.

Over half of the cases of argyria documented in the early 1900's were associated with silver nitrate use. (1) Silver nitrate is a caustic silver salt. It is not colloidal silver.

You can read Rosemary Jacob's story at: http://rosemaryjacobs.com/.

Another well publicized case of more recent vintage is that of Stan Jones. Stan Jones is a politician from Montana who acquired the condition of argyria by consuming extremely high quantities of a home-made colloidal silver. Stan brewed his home-made colloidal silver by using tap water and salt with a battery powered colloidal silver generator. He drank eight ounces or more of this product containing an unknown concentration of silver daily for at least two years. (102) This is far in excess of quantities that are usually used for therapeutic purposes. His source was also of dubious quality.

There have been additional recent cases of argyria reported. While the data is sketchy, it appears that there may be a half dozen or so cases reported. Fortunately, the number is extremely small compared to the number of individuals using silver products. It appears that those afflicted with argyria of recent origin used doses grossly in excess of amounts indicated for therapeutic effects. It also appears that they likely used products of unknown and questionable composition. They also consumed the substance over a long period of time, often years. Argyria from silver overdose is avoidable with good information, reliable silver products, and due diligence.

The amount of silver that must be consumed to cause argyria is not well understood. The risk factors for developing argyria depend on the dose of the silver product, the type of silver product, the duration of exposure, the route of exposure (i.e., ingestion, inhalation, or skin contact), and on the exposed individual's physiology and health.

There are reports that argyria has occurred in adults who were given 900 mg of silver orally over a period of one year. (1) There are also cases in the literature where 6.0

grams of silver nitrate administered orally and 6.3 grams of silver arsphenamine administered intramuscularly were known to produce argyria. (1) Another study estimated the minimal oral dose for producing argyria to be 25 to 50 grams taken over a 6 month period. (62) A single fatal dose is estimated to be 10 grams, although recovery from larger doses has been reported. (Note: This 10 gram figure is for silver nitrate which is significantly more toxic than colloidal silver.) (56)

Using the most conservative figure, 900 milligrams of silver corresponds to the silver content in 90 liters of 10 PPM colloidal silver. These doses are very large compared to the doses usually consumed by individuals using over the counter health food store colloidal silver products. Even with these quantities, risk of toxicity may be reduced by spreading the intake out over a period of time to allow the excretion mechanisms to keep up with intake.

Treating Argyria

Medical efforts to remove the skin pigmentation of argyria have not been very effective. There was one report posted on the internet claiming to have reversed argyria. This information has not been confirmed, but the claim merits investigation. The post is contained below in its entirety.

"The original post on the formula for Argyria Cured:

About two months ago, I was contacted by an individual with an amazing story:

This individual utilized 32 ounces of silver chloride daily for 2.5 years and cured a very late stage case of Nuerosyphilis. The silver chloride was produced in ten minute batches using the 3 nine-volt battery method of production with no controls. I have since spent quite some time on the phone with this individual.

The second part of this story:

By ingesting large amounts of a high concentration silver salt, the individual acquired argyria. It was likely a bit more severe than Stan Jones, but certainly not an aggravated condition like Rosemary Jacobs' agryria. It was bad enough to turn heads in a grocery store.

However, this individual didn't stop with eliminating his lethal condition. He also reversed the argyria.

Many have long discussed the possibility of using Vitamin E, Selenium, and other supplements with a cleansing program to reverse the condition, however, we've never seen someone actually accomplish it. It took six months of dedicated effort, but the individual's skin complexion returned to absolute normal.

Furthermore, the individual stopped taking the supplement program, resumed silver use, and his skin began to change once again. Whereby he resumed the supplementation, and the skin returned to normal.

Apparently, the silver build-up in the body when it reaches high enough levels to deposit visible silver in the skin is quite extensive. The process of removal is slow, but effective.

Furthermore, the individual actually had spirochetes in the eyes; the only thing that remains is slight scar tissue, and the individual, who was losing the use of the eyes, can see perfectly fine.

The list of symptoms with such an event is extensive. The individual was near liver failure, and within three months of initial silver use, was all but completely restored to full health. Fevers spiking 3-5 times daily, a chronic and severe lung infection, inflammation of the liver, shut down of the body's elimination systems, loss of reduction of cognitive ability, extreme and disabling fatigue are among the symptoms that fell to the power of this... Silver Chloride.

Obviously silver choride as a product is not equal to the superior isolated silver products. However, the question remains: Would consuming isolated silver have delivered enough actual silver content to the body to be effective in this case?

A Cure for Argyria: The Formula

3 Vitamin E 1000 mg 100% Natural d-alpha Tocopheryl (note that this can be a dangerous amount of Vitamin E)

1 Selenium 100mcg yeast free

2 vegetarian Vitamin C 1000 mg

1 teaspoon MSM organic

1 super potency Vitamin B 100,

1 teaspoon of Kelp powder:

Taken every morning with 2 16oz glasses of water, with close to a total of 3/4 of a gallon drinking water a day. ~ Jason" (104)

This post can be found at :
http://www.eytonsearth.org/forum/about7.html

30

Mechanism of Action - How it Works

It is believed that silver denatures proteins, enzymes in particular, of the target cell or organism by binding to reactive groups resulting in their precipitation and inactivation. Silver inactivates enzymes by reacting with the sulfhydryl groups to form silver sulfides. Silver also reacts with the amino, carboxyl, phosphate, and imidazole groups and diminish the activities of lactate dehydrogenase and glutathione peroxidase. Both gram positive and gram negative bacteria are in general affected by the oligodynamic effect of silver, but they can develop a silver resistance. The attachment of silver ions to one of these reactive groups on a protein results in the precipitation and denaturation of the protein. A good discussion of the current theories can be found in reference. (30)

Some researchers have noted that disinfection times with silver tend to be long and that silver forms reversible complexes with sulfhydryl and histidyl complexes of the cell surface and prevents the dehydrogenation process. In this model, silver presumably is responsible for protein denaturation on the cell surface resulting in inhibition of the growth of bacteria and viruses. It is the binding with sulfhydryl groups that interferes with bacterial respiration. This is a bacteriostatic effect and may be reversible if the silver is removed. (30)

Another effect is the affinity of silver to bind with DNA. It has been noted by several researchers that metals including silver do bind to DNA and thiol groups in bacteria and bacterial spores, and that reversible binding of bases occurs without aggregation or disruption of the double helix. Intercalation of silver can lead to increased stability of the double helix. The silver ions which bind to the bases and form cross links cause denaturation by displacing hydrogen bonds between the adjacent nitrogens, purines, and pyrimidines, thereby preventing replication. (30)(118)

It is believed that the interaction of silver with microorganisms is primarily with the proteins in the interstitial space when the silver ion concentration is low and with the membrane proteins and intracellular species when the silver ion concentration is high.

The diffusion of silver ions into mammalian tissues is self regulated by its intrinsic preference for binding to proteins as well as precipitation by the chloride ions in the environment. The affinity of silver ions to a large number of biologically important chemical moieties is also responsible for limiting its systemic action. (110)

In addition to the denaturation and precipitation of proteins, it is known that some silver compounds having low ionization or dissolution ability function effectively as antiseptics. Distilled water in contact with metallic silver becomes antibacterial, even though the dissolved concentration of silver ions is less than 100 PPB.

It is known that the efficacy of silver as an antimicrobial agent depends critically on the chemical and physical identity of the silver source. The silver source may be silver in the form of metal particles of varying sizes, silver as a sparingly soluble material such as silver chloride or silver as a highly soluble salt such as silver nitrate.

The efficiency of the silver also depends on the type of silver, whether it is the $Ag+$ ion or a complex species such as $AgCl_2$. The antibacterial efficacy of silver is determined by the type of silver, the concentration of the silver or silver compound, the type of microorganism, the surface area of the microorganism that is available for interaction with the silver, the concentration of the microorganism, and the specific mechanisms of deactivation. (111)(112)

There is evidence that pure silver does not possess germicidal or antibiotic properties. When molten silver is cooled in hydrogen, it does not possess antimicrobial activity. When cooled in air, silver exhibits antimicrobial activity. The implication is that surface oxidized silver is germicidal where pure silver is not. Researchers in the 1960s determined that the actual molecular formula of silver oxide is Ag_4O_4 with 50% of the silver atoms having a charge of +1 and the other 50% having a charge of +3. Experiments were performed in which Ag(II) and (III) disinfectants were shown to be 50-200 times as effective as Ag(I) compounds or metallic silver. Ag(III) works 240 times faster than Ag(I). Silver oxide is active against a wide variety of microbes. An *in vitro* experiment was performed in which 75% of AIDS viruses were killed in a solution of 10 PPM silver oxide. (116) (117)

Lok et. al., conducted studies on the oxidation states of silver nanoparticles and their antibacterial properties. "Partially (surface) oxidized silver nanoparticles have antibacterial activities, but zero-valent nanoparticles do not. The levels of chemisorbed Ag+ that form on the particle's surface, as revealed by changes in the surface plasmon resonance absorption during oxidation and reduction, correlate well with the observed antibacterial activities." (133)

It is reasonable to assume that silver colloidal particles have some degree of oxidation on their surface. The studies cited above establish that colloidal silver oxide is far more germicidal than pure metallic silver colloids.

It appears that colloidal silver does not remain in the blood stream for more than a few minutes once it is administered. It is believed that the reason silver does not remain in the blood for long is because it is rapidly protein bound and taken up by the reticuloendothelial system. The silver is deposited in the cells of the reticuloendothelial system, particularly in the liver and spleen, and to some extent in the lymph nodes. (46)

The research of Dr. Becker, et. al., (75) indicates that the small amounts of colloidal silver or silver ions generated in situ applied to wounds had a local antibiotic effect. That is, the silver and infectious germs had to be in direct contact. This is also the situation in petri dishes where in vitro germicidal tests are performed. In the case of Dr. Becker's research and Dr. Flick's silver bandages, the effect is a local one not a systemic one.

The reticuloendothelial cells are part of the immune system. They are the scavengers that consume foreign matter, cellular debris, invading germs, etc. One theory is that these cells regard the colloidal silver particles to be foreign material and consume them. The silver is then deposited in the cells. Since the same cells also ingest and absorb the invading germs, the invading germs and silver particles are brought into intimate contact. Once this occurs, the germicidal properties of the silver particles take their toll on the germs. The silver is apparently more toxic to prokaryotic cells and viruses than it is to human (eucaryotic) cells. It is not known how long the silver remains in the reticuloendothelial cells.

From studies with rabbits (44), it was observed that the rabbit was protected from the injection of an infectious agent twelve hours after an injection of electro colloidal silver. It is assumed that the silver would have been filtered out of the blood by then and would have either been mostly eliminated or stored in the tissues. Studies are needed to establish exactly how long colloidal silver remains in the blood in humans, exactly where it gets stored, how long it remains in storage, and how long after administration some antimicrobial effect can be observed.

It is known that silver is collected by the liver, excreted by the gall bladder, and eliminated in the feces. (63) Dr. Altman's experiments demonstrate that silver is eliminated primarily through the kidneys into the urine. (74) How much may be retained using a low dosage regimen and what effect that may have is unclear.

Another effect of administering colloidal silver internally is leukocytosis and elevated temperature. Leukocytosis is an elevation in the white blood cell count. It appears that the presence of the silver causes a stimulation of the immune system. The exact mechanism for this is not known. If colloidal silver is taken internally, the attending physician should consider taking before and after blood samples and observe the hematocrit, white cell count, and morphology. (44) Clinical studies in humans are needed to verify if this extrapolation from rabbit data is valid.

It is possible that there is a dosage range that is more than a homeopathic dose but less than an effective germicidal dose, in which a non-specific immune enhancing response is elicited. One model to look at is the homeopathic system. It is an empirical system which does not offer a (currently acceptable) scientific explanation for its underlying mechanisms. It uses dosages that are far below those that would be expected to provide germicidal effects. Everyone using colloidal silver should review the chapter on Homeopathy and understand its implications. One implication that cannot be overemphasized is that the Homeopathic Materia Medica also serves as a manual of symptomatic toxicology where large doses are used.

Many individuals using colloidal silver have reported a boost in energy and an improved sense of well being. Silver is used in ayurvedic medicine as a tonic or elixir to impart new energy to those debilitated by age or disease. The mechanism of this effect is unclear.

While the germicidal properties of silver are well known, its other effects are not as well understood. Dr. Becker noted that silver in combination with a DC microcurrent applied to wounds had an analgesic effect as well as a germicidal effect. He also noted accelerated wound healing. It appeared that the silver and microcurrent together have a synergistic effect.

Kenneth Wong and others at the University of Hong Kong recently investigated the wound-healing properties of silver nanoparticles. Wounds treated with silver nanoparticles healed in around 25 days, whereas it takes 29 days with common antibiotics, and 35 days with wounds left untreated. In addition to its antimicrobial properties, silver modifies cytokines – the enzymes involved in cell growth and movement – leading to reduced inflammation and an increased rate of healing. (106)

Pharmacodynamics

The observed physiological effects of colloidal silver and silver medicines in various forms include the following:

WBC Upregulation: Colloidal silver appears to increase the destructive action of white blood cells against pathogens by increasing the reactive oxygen species generated by the WBCs. (124)(125)

Lymphocytic Migration: The support of chemotaxis and tissue targeting of WBCs is implied by the inflammatory responses generated by the action of colloidal silver during infections. Herxheimer reactions modulate inflammatory cytokines which, in turn, can enhance lymphocytic migration. (125)(126)(127)

Leucocytosis: Leucocytosis (increases in the number of leucocytes) was observed by several investigators in the early 1900s. (44)(11) Bechhold confirmed that preliminary evidence was documented for oligodynamic silver to increase both RBC and WBC counts, but only after an initial hemolytic action took place that was transitory.

Hemolysis: Both early and recent investigators have noted a degree of transitory hemolysis after the administration of colloidal silver intravenously. (11)(44)(108)

Phagocytic Index: The phagocytic index is the average number of bacteria ingested by each phagocyte in an individual's blood after a mixture of the blood serum, bacteria, and phagocytes has been incubated. This implies an increased ability of phagocytes to engulf and destroy bacteria. A comprehensive retrospective text provided by Bechhold in 1919. The phagocytic index was increased by silver. (11)

Jarisch-Herxheimer Reactions: The Herxheimer reaction, also known as Jarisch-Herxheimer occurs when large quantities of toxins are released into the body as bacteria die. Typically the death of these bacteria and the associated release of endotoxins occurs faster than the body can remove the toxins via the natural detoxification process performed by the kidneys and liver. The accompanying symptoms include fever, chills, headache, nausea, muscle pain, skin lesions, and possibly a transitory immune system activation of coagulation. When extremely large doses of silver (i.e., ≥ 50 mg silver) are given, transitory hepatomegaly, and liver enzyme elevation can occur. While the Herxheimer reaction is usually associated with treatment of spirochete infections like syphilis and LYME disease, it may occur in other infections as well. (128)(129)(130)(131)

Germicidal and Antibiotic Activity: As noted above and below, colloidal silver demonstrates antimicrobial effects on pathogenic bacteria, viruses, fungi, and possibly some parasites like malaria.

The Germicidal Properties of Colloidal Silver

Colloidal Silver is regarded as a germicide. (8)(38)(39) (40)(72) These references indicate that it kills or inhibits many pathological organisms on contact. It can, therefore potentially be used as a topical antiseptic for application to cuts, scratches, wounds, burns, skin infections, etc. Potential methods of application include irrigation of minor wounds with a syringe, application to burns and skin infections with a wet dressing, application to burns with a spray bottle or wet dressing or in ointment form, irrigation of the nasal passages with a dropper or syringe, as a gargle to aid sore throats, etc.

In a letter published in the LANCET ("Electric Metallic Colloids and their Therapeutical Applications," Feb. 3, 1912) several studies were cited where colloidal silver prepared by chemical methods was used in vitro to kill cultures of B. Coli Communis, B. Tuberculous, Diplococcus Gonorrhea, various forms of staphylococcus and streptococcus, and others. The basic concentration was 500 PPM but effective results were also claimed for concentrations as low as 10 PPM and 5 PPM and in some cases even 1 PPM. (38)

An article published in the LANCET ("Experiments on the Germicidal Action of Colloidal Silver," Dec. 12, 1914) reports the results of an in vitro study of the effect of colloidal silver on cultures of typhoid bacillus. The colloidal silver was made by the chemical method and was tested in concentrations ranging from 5 PPM to 500 PPM. All of the typhoid bacillus was killed by 500 PPM colloidal silver within 30 minutes and within 2 hours by 10 PPM colloidal silver. 5 PPM colloidal silver was ineffective. (40)

An article published in the British Medical Journal ("The Bactericidal Action of Collosols of Silver and Mercury," Jan. 16, 1915) reports the results of bactericidal experiments of 500 PPM colloidal silver prepared by chemical methods on B. Coli Communis, B. Paratyphosis B., B. Parathphosis A., B. Typhosis, Staph. Pyogenes Aureus,   B. Anthracis, B. Pestis, B. Gaeriner, B. Danyes. In this study, no inhibition of growth was noted. Similar tests using silver nitrate at a concentration of 0.5 PPM indicated that the organisms were killed within 5 minutes. (41)

A letter from Larry C. Ford, M.D. ("Unpublished Letter," Larry C. Ford, M.D., University of California, Los Angeles, November 1, 1988) summarized a study using standard antimicrobial tests for disinfectants. It stated that the silver solutions tested were antibacterial for concentrations of 100,000 organisms per ml of streptococcus, Pyogenes, Staphylococcus Aureus, Neisseria Gonorrhea, Gardnerella Vaginalis, Salmonella Typhi, and other enteric pathogens and antifungal for Candida Albicans, Candida Alobata, and M. Furfur. The concentration of the silver preparations were unspecified in the letter.

Discovery Experimental and Development, Inc., a pharmaceutical company and Advantage Pharmaceuticals (8), has published several studies on their website. Their product is a 30 PPM protein stabilized colloidal silver made by a chemical process. They claim that their formulations have inhibited or have been lethal against HIV, C. Albicans, C. Neoformans, the spirochetes in LYME disease, E. Coli, S. Aureus, S. Neumonia, and P. Aeruginosa in in-vitro testing.

Here are some of the summaries:

1. A Letter from Willy Burgdorfer, Ph.D. at the National Institutes of Health 1995, claims that samples of colloidal silver at concentrations of 150 PPM and 15 PPM killed all of the LYME spirochete Borrelia Burgdorferi (B31) and the relapsing fever agent, B Hermsii (HS-1) within 24 hours.

2. A report issued by Earl E. Henderson, Ph.D., Professor, Temple University School of Medicine, 1995, describes the results of in vitro testing of silver proteins on the HIV-1 virus in the human lymphoblastoid cell line M57-3. This report claims that exposure to silver proteins from 10 to 100 PPM concentration inhibited the replication of HIV and a concentration of 1000 PPM eliminated the virus. Similarly, use of silver protein inhibited latency re-activation of the virus in human lymphoblastoid cells.

3. A report from Earl E. Henderson, Ph.D., Professor of Microbiology, Temple University School of Medicine, 1995, examines the effect of various concentrations of mild silver protein and aqueous colloidal silver on the replication of HIV-1 III B strain of the aids virus. These experiments show an in vitro inhibition on the replication of the HIV virus. The stronger concentrations produced greater results.

4. Another report describes the in vitro testing of the inhibition of the growth of drug resistant strains of Enterococcus by mild silver protein. The testing showed that moderate inhibition of growth occurred at concentrations of 1500 PPM but not at lower concentrations.

5. Another report examines the effect of silver proteins on the growth of E. Coli and S. Aureus. Growth of both was inhibited at concentrations of 1500 PPM but not at 150 PPM. Tests suggested that variable bactericidal results might be obtained at concentrations of 150 PPM and below.

6. A letter from Helen R. Buckley, Ph.D. at the Temple University School of Medicine, states that mild silver protein killed C. Albicans at concentrations between 46 and 93 PPM and inhibited their growth at concentrations between 0.7 and 1.4 PPM in vitro. C. Neoformans was killed by concentrations of 150-300 PPM and growth was inhibited by a concentration as low as 0.3 PPM in vitro. Candida Albicans and Cryptococcus Neoformans were killed by concentrations of 1500 PPM in vitro.

Daryl Tichy (71) contracted with the Department of Microbiology of Brigham Young University to conduct kill time studies with several bacteria species in the presence of the colloidal silver that he produced. The studies were conducted on standard strains of Salmonella Choleraesuis, Pseudomonas Aeruginosa, and Staphylococcus Aureus. The colloidal silver was demonstrated to be effective against these organisms. His colloidal silver was made by the electrocolloidal process but the concentration was not specified in the reports.

40

Dr. Ronald R. Gibbs (72) conducted a series of experiments on several brands and types of colloidal silver. He measured concentration, particle size, presence of dissolved solids, presence of "flocs" or clusters of silver particles, and germicidal properties. The least effective colloidal silver preparation had the same antimicrobial properties as tap water while the most effective was able to kill all bacteria colonies within 2.8 hours. The other products fell in between these two. He observed that the most effective products were those with the smallest colloidal particle sizes.

The conclusions from his research are (he presents data and graphs):

1. More concentrated colloidal silver (less diluted) preparations are more effective.

2. The colloidal silver products with the smaller particle sizes had the best germicidal properties.

3. In many cases bacteria diminished for a period of time after administration of colloidal silver, then overcame the effects of the colloidal silver and began growing again.

4. The addition of additional colloidal silver during the culture process enhanced the germicidal effect. Colloidal silver applied as a series of doses appears to be more germicidal than a single dose.

The summary is that colloidal silver products made by different manufacturers and different manufacturing methods have demonstrated germicidal properties. In addition, the germicidal properties vary from one product to another depending on a number of variables.

It is important to recognize that germicidal properties demonstrated in a petri dish do not necessarily indicate that the product will be effective as an oral or injected antibiotic.

American Silver, LLC, in the application for US Patent No. 7135195, reported in vitro kill data for their colloidal silver product against 56 common pathological disease microorganisms. The data was obtained by certified independent laboratories. The silver products had a concentration ranging from 2.5 to 10 parts per million. American Silver claimed that their product consisted of 97% metallic silver colloids and no ionic silver. All 56 species of microorganisms were killed in vitro. The list is included in the appendix.

Chambers, et. al., observed that the germicidal action of silver was related to the concentration of silver ions rather than from the type of silver from which the silver was delivered. They also observed that the germicidal properties of silver were not affected by pH but were interfered with by the presence of phosphate ions. (119)

Miller, et. al., observed that "Silver is taken up rapidly by fungus spores, so that germination can be completely inhibited after a contact time of 1 minute or less. Only mercury (I) and (II), and to a lesser extent copper, offer serious competition." (120)

Carr, et. al., performed in vitro antibacterial studies of silver sulfadiazine. They observed that 657 different types of bacteria from 22 different bacterial species were all inhibited by silver sulfadiazine. This may be the source of the widely circulated claim that colloidal silver cures 650 different diseases. Inhibiting bacteria in vitro is not curing a disease and silver sulfadiazine is not colloidal silver. (121)

Kim, et. al., investigated the antimicrobial properties of electrically generated silver nanoparticles. "The antimicrobial activity of Ag nanoparticles was investigated against yeast, Escherichia Coli, and Staphylococcus Aureus. In these tests, Muller Hinton agar plates were used and Ag nanoparticles of various concentrations were supplemented in liquid systems. As a result, yeast and E. Coli were inhibited at the low concentration of Ag nanoparticles, whereas the growth-inhibitory effects on S. Aureus were mild. The free-radical generation effect of Ag nanoparticles on microbial growth inhibition was investigated by electron spin resonance spectroscopy. These results suggest that Ag nanoparticles can be used as effective growth inhibitors in various microorganisms, making them applicable to diverse medical devices and antimicrobial control systems." (134)

Antibiotic Properties of Colloidal Silver

Silver was used as an antibiotic prior to the discovery of more modern antibiotics. A list of diseases, germs, and general conditions that colloidal silver has been used to treat in a historical context is listed in appendix A. This does not prove or even imply that colloidal silver should be used to treat these diseases today. Colloidal silver is not approved by the FDA for the treatment of any disease or medical condition at this time. Nevertheless, it has been and is being used by individuals who choose to regulate their own health care.

There are a couple of studies from the old medical literature that are of particular interest. They involve a product called Electrargol. Electrargol was a form of colloidal silver made from an electrical process. It is reported to have contained .04% silver. If this percentage is correct, this is equivalent to 400 mg of silver per liter of water or 400 PPM concentration of colloidal silver.

One article ("Electric Metallic Colloids and their Therapeutical Applications," THE LANCET, Jan. 13, 1912) (37) discusses the uses of Electrargol. The author of this article is of the opinion that the electrically manufactured colloids are so superior to the chemically produced ones that they alone should be considered for use. The information in this article is useful for comparative purposes.

In summary, Electrargol was used in infective states of septicemia and pyemia for which from 5 to 20 cc was injected into a muscle or a major vein. In cases of local infections such as epididymitis, bubo, mammary abscess, etc., injections are made directly into the lesion in addition to the constitutional treatment. Colloidal silver was also injected into the spinal canal, the serous cavities, and applied locally. Colloidal silver was also used in the treatment of the lungs and pleura with dramatic results. This author claims that there was no pain, irritation or toxic reactions, and that there should be no hesitation in injecting 3 to 5 cc intramuscularly. Numerous publications are cited for their case histories from other physicians verifying these positive results.

Another major article on Electrargol is "Colloidal Silver in Sepsis," Journal of the American Association of Obstetricians and Gynecologists, Jan , 1916. (44) This paper observes that Electrargol has two therapeutic actions. First, it is a powerful germicide. In one test, colonies of virulent streptococci were sprayed with Electrargol and cultures transplanted to fresh media. Those that came into contact with Electrargol showed no growth. The second effect is leukocytosis. Rabbits were injected with 1/2 cc of Electrargol (200 mcg. of silver) and the white cell count taken before and after. The white cells raised from 6000 to 10-13,000; the polymorphonuclear leukocytes from 50 or 60 percent to 80 to 90 percent. Twelve hours after the injection there appeared a slight leukolysis (7,000-6,600) but after twenty four hours the high leukocytosis always appeared.

Experiments were performed in vivo in rabbits using Electrargol and streptococcus organisms. In the control rabbit the temperature was 96, leukocyte count 6600, and polymorphonuclear leukocytes 34%. The control was then injected with 1/2 cc virulent streptococci intraperitoneally. The next day, the control was quiet, temperature 96.4, leukocyte count 15,000 with 76% polymorphonuclear leukocytes. After three days, the control was restless, leukocyte count 17,000, temperature 102, blood cultures show streptococci. The Rabbit died after 7 days.

In the treated rabbit, the temperature was 96.5, leukocyte count 8000 with 43% polymorphonuclears. The treated rabbit was injected with 3 cc Electrargol, then twelve hours later it was injected with 1/2 cc of the same virulent streptococci. The next day the leukocyte count was 10,000 with 60 percent polymorphonuclear leukocytes. After 48 hours, the blood cultures did not show any growth. After 72 hours, the rabbit was lively and showed no symptoms of illness. The leukocyte count was 7,000. The rabbit remained well.

In the same paper, the authors reviewed some of their own clinical cases with humans. The authors noted that their patients experienced a temperature rise three to five hours after administration of the Electrargol. They believe that this was caused by the release of toxins from bacteria that were destroyed by the Electrargol.

Several case histories were reported. In one, a severe case of septicemia was treated with 5 cc of Electrargol intravenously. Within 3 days his temperature was reduced and the symptoms were subsiding. This patient recovered fully. Another patient with severe septicemia received intravenous injections of 5 cc Electrargol at approximate 48 hour intervals for a total of 3 treatments. She recovered and was discharged ten days later. Another case of severe septicemia received two injections of Electrargol at 24 hour intervals. After 48 hours her temperature and other symptoms had returned to normal. It should be noted that without antibiotics, cases of this severity usually resulted in death. Also, the victims were often women and the cause of septicemia was either from an infected injury or childbirth.

If one assumes that a linear interpolation from the body weight of a rabbit to that of a human, a point of reference might be the administration of 10 mg of silver for a 160 pound adult to produce an observed leukocytosis. In some anecdotal reports, individuals self administered approximately 1 mg of silver and obtained relief from symptoms of colds, flu, mumps, etc.

Another paper ("Some Recent Observations on Sprue," The British Medical Journal, Nov. 15, 1913) (39), discusses the course and prognosis of Sprue. Collosol Argentum as the treatment of choice. (It was silver and silver oxide in colloidal form at a standard concentration of 500 PPM.) The author states that B. Coli Communis is killed in 10 seconds by this preparation and that no microbe is known that is not killed in six minutes. His dosage was 1 or 2 or more drachmas (about 7.5 ml) two or three times daily. In 76 to 118 hours stools would lose their frothiness and show appropriate bulk even in cases where the temperature was over 101 F and death was anticipated.

Another paper ("Collosol Argentum and its Ophthalmic uses," British Medical Journal, Jan 16, 1915) (42), discusses several cases of treatment of eye disorders with Collosol

Argentum. (This is colloidal silver from chemical sources at a concentration of 500 PPM.) The author states that Collosol Argentum is far superior than his other remedies (which include silver nitrate, yellow oxide of mercury, etc.) in the treatment of eye infections and corneal ulcers. This also applies to interstitial keratitis (treated with drops three times per day) and blepharitis. He also used Collosol Argentum for the treatment of dacrosystitis after syringing out the sac with saline and for wounds and conjunctivitis.

Another paper ("A Case of Puerperal Septicemia Successfully Treated with Intravenous Injections of Collosol Argentum," Lancet, Feb. 16, 1916) (43) describes a very serious case of sepsis following childbirth. The patient did not respond to any of the treatments available (which did not include antibiotics). Intravenous injections of Collosol Argentum (500 PPM silver) in the amount of 20 cc every 48 hours were given. Dramatic improvement was noted on the day following each injection and no undesirable side effects were noted.

Discovery Experimental and Development, Inc., (8) has published several case studies on their website. LYME disease is a very dangerous and stubborn disease that often resists antibiotic treatment. Their protocol can be used as a point of reference in designing research protocols for similar serious infectious diseases. In some cases their treatment protocol calls for a quantity of silver intake equal to about 5% of the most conservative silver intake that has been known to produce argyria in adults. Still, if it is a choice between an otherwise incurable infection and a risk of argyria, one has to take into perspective the tradeoff between other antibiotics and their side effects.

Dr. J. Cardot, M.D., in a letter published on the Internet (8) claims successful treatment of over 50 cases of viral pneumonia with 30 PPM silver protein at a dosage of 1 tbs t.i.d. (three times per day) for a duration of between 4 and 30 days depending on the severity of the case. This corresponds to a total cumulative dose ranging from 5.4 mg to 40.5 mg. He claims similar success with other infections including ear infections in children, infectious fibromyalgia,

Sjorgen's syndrome, rheumatoid arthritis with synovial fluid infections, systemic candida albicans, Staph infections, gingivitis, LYME disease (Borrelia burgdorferi), HIV, ringworm, psoriasis, genital herpes, and herpes zoster. (8)

There is a clear and definite history of the apparently successful use of many forms of silver as an antibiotic in old medical literature and in current anecdotal accounts. It seems that the question is not one of determining "if" colloidal silver is an antibiotic but in performing the necessary research and development and clinical trials to determine the relative effectiveness of different types of colloidal silver, the best way to manufacture the product, and the best way to apply it clinically. Then there is the question of whether colloidal silver would be better than or inferior to standard antibiotics or other alternatives for particular situations.

In a recent clinical study, three patients with HIV were treated with a 40 PPM, 400 PPM, and 1500 PPM mild silver protein. The initial protocol involved orally administered MSP in increasing dosages for 30 days followed by a series of intravenous infusions. Oral MSP was continued throughout the treatment. The infusion consisted of 120 ml of MSP of 40, 400, and 1500 PPM concentration in a carrier solution which included dimethyl sulfoxide (DMSO). The infusion was delivered over a period of 2 to 3 hours.

One subject experienced weakness and severe myalgia after administration of a treatment at 1500 PPM. This was regarded to be a Herxheimer reaction. This patient also experienced a severe reduction in red blood cell count and a drop in hemoglobin levels after the 1500 PPM treatment. It was concluded that 1500 PPM MSP administered intravenously was probably toxic. This patient's HIV viral count was initially 750,000 RNA copies/ml. After 60 days, no HIV viruses were detectable. All three patients experienced a dramatic and rapid reduction in viral loads. (108)

Rendin, et. al., used colloidal silver oxide to treat 88 patients with peptic ulcer. Within 6 weeks, all cases except one were healed. Subsequently, it was discovered that peptic ulcers are caused by an infection of Helicobacter pylori. (122)

Silver Applied as a Topical Germ Killer

Silver has a long history of use as a topical germ killer. Silver foil, sutures and implantable devices have been used in medicine since the late 1800's. These dressings were used extensively until just after World War II, and were listed in the Physician's Desk Reference until 1955, when the use of antibiotics became widespread.

In the early 1970's, Drs. Becker, Marino, and Spadaro, of the Veterans Administration Hospital in Syracuse, New York, pioneered the study of silver-coated fabrics for the treatment of complex bone infections. Subsequently, Dr. A. B. Flick began developing broader clinical applications for silver nylon fabrics in treating wounds and burns. Dr. Flick founded Argentum Medical, LLC to manufacture silver plated fabric bandages for wound and burn care. Argentum Medical was the first manufacturer to obtain FDA and other regulatory approvals for silver products for these applications. Subsequently, at least a half dozen other companies have started producing silver containing bandage products.

The popularity of colloidal silver as an alternative germ fighter has drawn the attention of doctors, researchers, regulators, and a variety of corporations. The result has been twofold. One result is new research and the introduction of new products. The other is the attempt to suppress silver products as a potential competitor of high value anti-microbial drugs.

The new products include soaps, cosmetics, toothpaste, clothing, and appliances. Samsung has introduced a refrigerator and laundry washing machine that uses silver coated surfaces to eliminate odor causing bacteria. Adidas and Polartec have licensed silver coated nylon fabric to incorporate antimicrobial silver into athletic and outdoor clothing. Brooks Sports sells silver impregnated socks, caps, and shirts. ARC Outdoors produces silver impregnated antimicrobial socks for the military, Wal-Mart, Cabela's, and Bass ProShops. SmartSilver is a brand of odor-eliminating underwear, stocking caps, and gloves that kills bacteria on contact.

The Development of Silver Resistance in Bacteria

Appendix A lists 6 microorganisms that have strains that are known to possess silver resistance.

Some organisms have mechanisms to evade the toxic effects of metals. Several species of bacteria have been shown to possess a copper resistance gene. Also, silver resistant microorganisms isolated from the soil in silver mines have been shown to actually accumulate silver at the astonishing concentration of 23 mg of silver per gram of dry weight. Life is indeed diverse and adaptable. (30)

Resistance to silver compounds as determined by bacterial plasmids and genes has been defined by molecular genetics. Silver resistance conferred by the Salmonella plasmid pMGH100 involves nine genes in three transcription units. (135)

Given that bacteria are capable of transferring genetic material from one organism to another and that silver resistant genes exist in nature, increased use of silver products will inevitably lead to silver resistant pathogens. This has not happened to any recognized degree yet because silver containing antibiotics were nearly entirely abandoned with the introduction of modern antibiotics. There are, however, many serious pathogens with multiple antibiotic resistances as a result of over use of antibiotic drugs.

Perhaps we will be smart enough to not make the same mistake with silver?

Effective Dosage - How much is required?

Unfortunately, there is no definitive answer to this question. Again there is only information that can serve as clues or guidelines from which a "guess" can be made. Again, this is not intended to be a recommendation for use, but as correlative information for academic or research purposes.

There are a lot of variables in colloidal silver products. Some products are stabilized by proteins or organic acids. Some products are manufactured by chemical precipitation and others by electrical methods. Modern experimental methods may incorporate light, lasers, gamma rays, microwaves, and ultrasound, often in conjunction with complex organic chemicals. Those made by electrical methods may vary significantly as the manufacturing parameters change.

In the previous reference to Electrargol, the authors indicated that a typical treatment in humans might include injecting from 5 to 20 cc into a muscle or a major vein and that physicians should have no hesitation in injecting 3 to 5 cc intramuscularly. At a concentration of 400 PPM, 3 cc's contain 1.2 mg. of silver, 5 cc's contain 2 mg of silver, and 20 cc's contain 8 mg of silver. In several cases, the injections of 5 cc's were repeated at 24 or 48 hour intervals for a total of two or three treatments, if needed. (37)(44)

In comparison to these numbers, the DEDI protocol for treating LYME disease (8) recommends the oral consumption of 1.5 liters of 30 PPM mild silver protein (over a period of one month, and up to twice that amount for some cases) or more depending on symptoms. This represents 45 to 90 milligrams of silver. This is from 5% to 10% of the dose that produced argyria in an adult in our most conservative example. (1)

I have heard anecdotal reports of individuals consuming 1 liter of 1 PPM colloidal silver to knock out the common cold. This represents a cumulative dose of 1 mg of silver. Most, but not all of them, reported positive results. In equivalent silver content this is comparable to the 5 cc injection of Electrargol that was used to treat septicemia in humans. This dose is approximately three times the EPA RFD for daily silver consumption from natural sources.

Dr. J. Charcot, M.D. (8) claims to have successfully treated over 50 cases of viral pneumonia using 30 PPM protein bound colloidal silver (produced by chemical precipitation) at doses of 1 tbs three times per day for a duration of between 4 and 30 days. This corresponds to a total silver consumption of between 5.4 mg and 40.5 mg for a 160 pound adult.

This data is useful for crude comparisons only. Human studies on effectiveness are needed to give a definitive answer regarding how much is safe and how much is an effective treatment for different infections and for different silver products.

In pharmacology, there is an effective dose and a lethal dose for any particular drug. The ratio of the lethal dose (for 50% of the test population) to the effective dose (for 50% of the test population) is called the therapeutic index. It is desirable to have a therapeutic index as large as possible in order to be able to administer effective therapy without causing harm. There isn't enough data to determine a therapeutic index. However, using animal and human data and extrapolating, one could make a rough estimate of a therapeutic index of between 200 and 10,000 for colloidal silver. This is using 10 grams as the lethal dose and between 1 and 50 milligrams as the effective dose.

It is not known if the reticuloendothelial cells retain the silver indefinitely or manage to excrete some or all of it over time. It is possible that if they do retain it, one course of treatment may afford some permanent enhancement to ones resistant to infection. If this is so, repetitive dosing may not be necessary.

The Homeopathic Materia Medica is, in addition to a catalog of remedies, an excellent reference on the symptomatic toxicology of a large number of natural substances including silver. See reference (51).

The dosage information presented above was taken from information on colloidal silver produced by electrical methods and, in some cases, from information of mild silver protein, MSP. Information from Natural Immunogenics Corp. and other manufacturers suggests that much smaller doses are effective and more appropriate. Their dosage recommendations fall well below the EPA reference dose for silver consumption. Their opinion is that their exceptionally small colloidal particle sizes make the silver more effective so that less is required. Controlled human clinical trials are needed for clarification and refined understanding.

An additional note on dosage is that several manufacturers have suggested that frequent doses, i.e. every two to three hours, may be more effective than large doses. This is reasonable because all currently available information suggests that silver remains in the blood for only a very short time. It is presumed that the ideal way to administer colloidal silver for a systemic antibiotic effect is by intravenous drip. This is certainly not something anyone should do at home especially with home made colloidal silver.

Silver & Electro-Colloidal Silver in Wound Treatment

The book The Body Electric by Robert O. Becker, M.D. and Gary Selden, discusses the pioneering work done by Robert O. Becker and others on the role of electricity in healing and tissue regeneration. They devote an entire chapter on the role of silver in this process. Chapter 8, The Silver Wand, summarizes their results using silver electrodes and very small electric currents.

"In preliminary tests we found that silver electrodes, when made electrically positive, would kill all types of bacteria in a zone about a half inch in diameter." (7)

"Our preliminary observations turned out to be right. Silver at the positive pole killed or deactivated every type of bacteria without side effects, even with very low currents." (7)

"We were certain that it was the silver ions that did the job, rather than the current, when we found that the silver impregnated culture medium killed new bacteria placed in it, even after the current was switched off." (7)

Note: The application of a positive direct current to a silver electrode resembles one of the popular processes of making colloidal silver. From the level of currents that they used (100-200 nanoamperes per square centimeter), the concentration of silver or silver chloride colloids or silver ions would have to be quite low.

Before the antibiotic era, metal wire and metal foil were used in dressing wounds apparently with good effect. The amount of silver colloids or ions coming off the surface of the silver by diffusion would, also, have to be quite small.

While Dr. Becker was convinced that the antibacterial effects were due to the silver, more recent research has demonstrated that a direct current, in the range Dr. Becker was using, is able to kill the AIDS virus and other pathogenic organisms. Perhaps the electric current and silver have a synergistic effect. In addition to the antibacterial effects of silver, they discovered that the silver appeared to work in conjunction with the electric current to induce de-differentiation of cells and accelerate tissue repair and regeneration.

"We may only have scratched the surface of positive silver's medical brilliance. Already it's an amazing tool. It stimulates bone-forming cells, cures the most stubborn infections of all kinds of bacteria, and stimulates healing in skin and other soft tissues. We don't know whether the treatment can induce healing in other parts of the body, but the possibility is there, and there may be other marvels latent in this magic caduceus. Just before our research group was disbanded, we studied malignant fibro sarcoma cells (cancerous fibroblasts) and found that electrically injected silver suspended their runaway mitosis. Most important of all, the technique makes it possible to produce large numbers of dedifferentiated cells, overcoming the main problem of mammalian regeneration the limited number of bone marrow cells that dedifferentiate in response to electrical current alone. Whatever its precise mode of action may be, the electrically generated silver ion can produce enough cells for human blastemas; it has restored my belief that full regeneration of limbs, and perhaps other body parts, can be accomplished in humans." (7)

Becker further states, in reference (57), that the combined application of silver and low level electric currents cause de-differentiation of fibroblasts. Fibroblasts are a common cell type which could contribute significantly to healing and regeneration when converted to other cell types. It is important to note that both the silver and low level direct current were required to produce this effect.

In reference (58), the author discusses the chemical characteristics of silver in human biological systems. Silver does deactivate at least some human enzymes. However, this effect is generally not seen in vivo (in living organisms) because the silver readily binds to serum proteins. Silver also interacts with cellular DNA. Silver binds strongly to the DNA replacing the H bonds of the DNA double helix. The new helix has a much larger diameter. Silver also causes a compaction of the DNA molecule. These effects are reversible when the silver is removed. What this means is unclear but may have something to do with the dedifferentiation of cells.

The research of Dr. Becker and others established that all types of bacteria were killed within about a half inch around the silver electrode when a current of 100-200 nanoamperes per square centimeter of electrode was applied. Under these conditions, low concentrations of colloidal silver and colloidal silver chloride particles would be created on the spot and diffused directly into the tissues, and into contact with any microorganisms in the area. (7)

This research suggests that this principle might be used in the treatment of superficial or otherwise accessible infections and infectious lesions. An abscess could have a silver wire or needle inserted directly into it and a small electrical current applied. A skin infection could be covered with a piece of silver foil or silver coated fabric and a small current applied. A puncture or surgical wound could have a piece of silver placed into the wound and a small current applied with the intent of preventing infection and accelerating healing. Silver wires could be easily removed after healing was complete. A body part could be immersed in water or normal saline and current applied through a silver electrode. The result would be colloidal particles of silver attaching to the surface of the skin or permeating the mass of a boil or lesion.

In Dr. Becker's work, the current level used in the electro diffusion of silver colloids into tissue was in the range of 100 to 300 nanoamperes per square centimeter of silver electrode. This situation applies where the silver is in direct contact with the tissue. If a water bath is used and the silver is not in direct contact with the tissue, the tissue area would be used rather than the silver electrode area in computing current density.

Dr. Becker, et. al., determined that tissue electrolysis (tissue damage or destruction) occurred when a voltage of 1.1 VDC was applied directly to the tissues. They therefore limited their applied voltage to 0.9 VDC or less. In contrast, in the use of iontophoresis, the current may run from 1/2 to 10 milliamperes depending upon the electrode area and configuration. These current levels are much higher than Becker's applications and cannot be expected to have the same effect.

In electrosurgery, where electrolysis is used to destroy small areas of tissues such as moles, warts, skin cancers, etc., direct currents of a few milliamperes are used, but through a smaller surface area such as a needle. If silver needles were used, silver colloids would be generated and diffused directly into the tissues. It is reasonable to assume that silver diffused into the necrotic tissue by this process would assist in preventing the development of infections.

When estimating electrode surface area and current density, it is probably better to err toward smaller currents rather than larger ones. There does not appear to be well defined threshold zone in which tissue healing is stimulated by small currents, but not large ones. The diffusion of silver particles will take place at all current densities. It is a little faster with larger currents, but that appears to be unnecessary.

A successful clinical application of this principle is described in reference. (60) Open wounds were treated by applying silver impregnated nylon cloth directly to the wound and applying a 900 millivolt DC source to the cloth. Dr. Flick concluded "The use of electrical silver iontophoresis is considered an extremely valuable tool in the treatment of both bone and soft tissue infections. Wounds are sterilized and granulation tissue stimulated with this technique. There were no significant complications noted."

The antimicrobial, healing, and analgesic effects of silver bandages, and/or silver bandages with a small electrical current applied, are local and not systemic by intention. While the research referenced here focused on this local effect of bandages with or without electric current applied, there are other informal reports of farmers and veterinarians using liquid colloidal silver to irrigate wounds and abscesses in animals, and of dentists using colloidal silver to irrigate oral infections as in abscesses, extractions, etc.

A relatively new company, Argentum Research, Inc., has introduced a line of silver plated bandages. These products are FDA approved and backed by clinical research and testing. These products have been shown to be antibacterial and antifungal to all species tested to date that are known to infect human and animal wounds. This includes Staphylococcus Aureus (i.e., MRSA, or Methicilln Resistant Staph Aureus) or Escherichia Faecalis (i.e., VRE, or Vancomycin Resistance Escherichia Faecalis). They have also been discovered to offer a significant reduction in pain and inflammation as well.

Following the success of Argentum Research, several companies have introduced silver bandages, dressings, and related products. The competitors include Band-Aid® by Johnson & Johnson and Acticoat® by Westaim Biomedical.

Iontophoresis using Silver and Copper

Iontophoresis as a therapeutic modality has been in use by several health care professions including medical, osteopathic, naturopathic and chiropractic physicians, and physical therapists since the early 1900's. It fell into disuse because it is messy and time consuming and, for many of its former applications, pharmaceutical products were promoted as an alternative.

There are some applications, however, where it excels. Iontophoresis is being rediscovered as a noninvasive modality with fewer risks and contraindications than its pharmaceutical alternatives. It is finding widespread use by physical therapists, chiropractors, and allopathic physicians as well.

Iontophoresis is the process of diffusing ions into human tissue with the aid of a low voltage direct current. Some of the applications involve the use of metal ions, such as silver or copper, for the inhibition of skin infections and the diffusion of drugs directly into tissues rather than administering them systemically. Copper iontophoresis has specifically been used to treat athlete's foot and other fungal infections. Other applications are the diffusion of anti-inflammatory drugs into painful or swollen tissues.

Iontophoresis uses ions as the therapeutic agent rather than colloids. In the case of copper iontophoresis, copper sulfate is usually the conductive medium used. If silver were used, silver nitrate might be employed but would have to be very dilute since it is caustic. The use of silver nitrate should only be used under a physician's direction. One could use distilled water or a mild saline solution with silver rather than a solution of silver ions. The result would be that silver or silver chloride colloidal particles would leave the positive silver electrode and attach themselves to the skin surface being treated. This would not be caustic to the skin and would have germicidal effects. The diffusion of copper ions into the surface of the skin can cause a light blue-green discoloration which wears off. The use of silver could also cause a discoloration which might be more persistent since silver so readily binds to proteins.

A typical setup for an iontophoresis treatment consists of a low voltage DC power source, a container with an appropriate ionic solution in it, an electrode to supply additional ions, and a dispersive pad attached to the body. The dispersive pad consists of a sponge saturated with a conductive solution, a stainless steel electrode, and a rubber strap to attach the electrode assembly to the skin. Assembled electrodes for iontophoresis therapy and the appropriate power sources can be purchased from physical therapy suppliers.

For more details on iontophoresis therapy, consult references (53), (54), and (55).

Modern Scientific Homeopathy

Classical Homeopathy was developed before the age of modern scientific tools. Subsequently, Homeopaty fell out of favor and became relegated to "fringe" status. More subsequently, modern science is beginning to crack the misunderstandings of science and medicine. The contemporary book, Homeopathy: A Frontier In Medical Science, gives a good overview of new developments in this area.

A controversy was generated when French researcher J. Benveniste published a report in Nature describing his research with high dilutions of antigens and their ability to cause an allergic reaction, although there were theoretically no molecules of the original antigen remaining. He was published because of his high standing in the scientific community and because his research was of the highest professional quality. Without saying it in specific words, he was describing the process of making high potency homeopathic agents and validating their ability to act effectively. When the editors realized what had happened, they sent debunkers to tear apart and discredit his work. He was subsequently discredited, harassed, and had his funding and support withdrawn. The scientific community was appalled at the treatment of Benveniste. Good scientists are pragmatic people who don't tolerate bullshit and look for opportunities to sit down and determine what the truth is, by a rigorous process of testing the divergent concepts and theories. In reality, progress is often held up by decades, even today, by the victory of theory, prejudice, money and politics over facts and truth. A full account of this affair can be found in the book The Memory of Water (66).

Nevertheless, the cat was out of the bag, so to speak, and those with the inclination are continuing this line of investigation. This line of research may eventually explain why very small quantities of substances, like silver, can project an affect that appears to be far out of proportion to their concentration.

Silver in Classical Homeopathy

The anecdotal reports for the effectiveness of colloidal silver are numerous and sometimes dramatic. It is possible that some of the benefits that have been reported result from properties other than germicidal or immune enhancing.

In Homeopathy, the proving of a remedy consisted of taking a group of healthy individuals and giving them large doses of the remedy in question and observing the symptoms that develop from the overdosing. They then dilute the remedy and use the dilution to treat individuals who presented similar symptoms without exposure to the substance.

These "provings" are catalogued in the <u>Homeopathic Materia Medica and Repertory</u> by William Boericke, M.D., Sett Dey & Co., Calcutta, 1976. The repertory serves as a huge catalog for the correlation of symptoms with the appropriate remedy. It is also a catalog of the symptomatic toxicology for a large number of natural substances, including silver.

The following is quoted from <u>Materia Medica and Repertory</u> under the remedy for Argentum Metallicum (silver):

"Emaciation, a gradual drying up, desire for fresh air, dyspnoea, sensation of expansion and left-sided pains are characteristic. The chief action is centered on the articulations and their component elements, bones, cartilages, and ligaments. Here the small blood vessels become closed up or withered and carious affections result. They come on insidiously, lingering, but progress. The larynx is also a special center for this drug.

Mental. - Hurried feeling; time passes slowly; melancholy.

Head. - Dull paroxysmal neuralgia over left side, gradually increasing and ceasing suddenly. Scalp very tender to touch. Vertigo, with intoxicated feeling, on looking at running water. Head feels empty, hollow. Eyelids red and thick. Exhausting coryza, with

62

sneezing. Pain in facial bones. Pain between left eye and frontal eminence.

Throat. - Raw, hawking, gray, jelly-like mucus, and throat sore on coughing. Profuse and easy morning expectoration.

Respiratory. - Hoarseness Aphonia. Raw, sore feeling when coughing. Total loss of voice of professional singers. Larynx feels sore and raw. Easy expectoration, looking like boiled starch. Feeling of raw spot near supra sternal fossa. Worse from use of voice. Cough from laughing. Hectic fever at noon. On reading aloud, must hem and hawk. Great weakness of chest; worse left side. Alteration in timbre of voice. Pain in left lower ribs.

Back. - Severe backache; must walk bent, with oppression of chest.

Urine. - Diuresis. Urine profuse, turbid, sweet odor. Frequent urination. Polyuria.

Extremities. - Rheumatic affections of joints, especially elbow and knee. Legs weak and trembling, worse descending stairs. Involuntary contractions of fingers, partial paralysis of forearm; writer's cramp. Swelling of ankles.

Male. - Crushed pain in testicles. Seminal emissions, without sexual excitement. Frequent micturation with burning.

Female. - Ovaries feel too large. Bearing-down pain. Prolapse of womb. Eroded spongy cervix. Leucorrhaea foul, excoriating. Palliative in scirrhus of uterus. Pain in left ovary. Climacteric haemorrhage. Sore feeling throughout abdomen; worse by jarring. Uterine disease with pain in joints and limbs.

Modalities. -Worse from touch, towards noon. Better in open air, cough at night when lying down (opposite Hyoscy.)

Relationship. - Antidotes: Mercur.; Puls.

Compare: Selen.; Alum.; Platina; Stannum; Ampelopsis. (Chronic hoarseness in scrofulous patients.)

Dose. - Sixth trituration and higher. Not too frequent repetition."

A Homeopathic physician would regard these symptoms as an indication to administer silver as a remedy. Remember, however, that excess dosage of silver could potentially cause these same symptoms.

Colloidal Silver is not prepared in the same manner as Homeopathic drugs and is therefore not a Homeopathic drug. However, the process of making a colloid has some similarities to trituration and the Homeopathic information may be useful for comparative purposes. The sixth trituration, 6X, would be roughly equivalent to one part per million concentration.

One must consider that colloidal silver may work in a similar fashion to a homeopathic remedy. If this is the functional mechanism, a few drops under the tongue would be the only dosage required. Also, more dilute concentrations may be more effective than larger ones.

To test colloidal silver for its homeopathic effects, take a sample of your colloidal silver and dilute it into four samples having concentrations of 10 PPM, 1 PPM, 0.1 PPM, 0.01 PPM, and 0.001 PPM with distilled water. These dilution's correspond to the Homeopathic potencies of 5X, 6X, 7X, 8X, and 9X respectively.

Then look for a patient with these symptoms:

Inflammation and congestion of lungs, runny nose & raw throat, hoarseness and loss of voice, joint pain, cramps, headaches, worse on left side. Consult the symptom profile above for a more complete picture of the 'silver' patient.

The dose for this test is 3 to 5 drops under the tongue. Start with the most dilute sols and progress to the less dilute ones if they show no effect. If this experiment is effective, relief of symptoms should be noted in minutes. Repetition of the dose should be infrequent. This evaluation is entirely subjective. In the homeopathic belief system the .001 PPM suspension should be more powerful than the 1 PPM suspension. While the method of preparation is different, 10 PPM corresponds to 5x, 1 PPM corresponds to 6x, .1 PPM corresponds to 7x, etc.

These small highly dilute doses do not represent an appreciable hazard of silver toxicity.

Ayurvedic Properties of Silver

The traditional Ayurvedic Medicine of India used specially prepared metals and oxides of metals for therapeutic purposes.

"Silver is cooling though sour, and is used to cool the mind, emotions, and body in conditions such as neuritis and neuralgia, inflammations of the mucous membranes, diseases of the reproductive system, and lunacy. It is also an aphrodisiac and is useful in cases of debility. Even in ionic form, silver is fundamentally non-toxic to human cells, even more so than Gold." (6)

"Contrary to gold, it (silver) is cool by nature and therefore it is used for the treatment of excessive 'Pitta' present in the body. It can also be used for the treatment of 'Vata' ailments; however, silver should be used with caution for the treatment of 'Kapha' constitution people. Silver strengthens the muscles and increases the stamina and is also helpful for emaciation, chronic fever, weakness after fever, digestive problems, heartburn, acidity, hyperactivity of the gall bladde,r and problems of menstrual bleeding. Its ash (Bhasma) may be used for the treatment of inflammatory heart diseases, liver, and spleen disorders. Silver water (prepared by the same method as gold water) is used for increasing the strength of muscles and enhancing stamina." (101)

Colloidal Silver is not prepared in the manner of Ayurvedic medicines. This information is presented for comparative purposes only.

Colloidal Silver as a Food Supplement

While silver is found in the human body and some foodstuffs, the need, or lack of need, for silver in human nutrition has not been scientifically established.

In reviewing some of the old medical literature, I found references to silver being concentrated in the thyroid gland and tonsils in particular and other organs in general. (67) It was noted that silver had a stimulating effect on the growth of watercress and on the nicotine secreting hairs of the tobacco plant. In edible fungi, silver is concentrated in amounts of up to 0.2% of dry weight. (67)

Given that some animal and plant organs and tissues concentrate silver, it is possible that it may have some metabolic role. Scientists have, so far, not identified what that role, if any, is.

The Manufacture of Colloidal Silver

Historically, several methods of making silver and other metallic colloids have been tried. Mechanical grinding to produce extremely small silver particles was not very successful because the particle size was too large. Chemical precipitation, that is, the addition of a reducing agent to a silver salt, usually silver nitrate, with the resulting precipitate forming colloidal particles is another method. Many of the pre-1938 silver compounds and some of the modern products use some form of this method. There are some drawbacks to this method. No chemical reaction goes to 100% completion and some of the reactants remain. Thus, there will be traces of silver nitrate and a quantity of whatever the reducing agent was used. The other methods are electrical, either a cathodic process or one of several configurations of electric arc. The method described here is the cathodic method because it is the simplest and safest and requires the least amount of equipment and materials.

There is some argument and discussion among colloidal silver manufacturers about whether a product is "colloidal" or "ionic" and which is most desirable. An ion is an atom or molecule which has lost or gained one or more electrons, giving it a positive or negative electrical charge. Cations are positively charged ions, formed when an atom loses electrons in a reaction, forming an "electron hole." Cations are the opposite of anions, since cations have fewer electrons than protons.

Water molecules are formed from two atoms of hydrogen and one of oxygen in a polar covalent bond. There is an electrical charge on water molecules because of the uneven sharing of the electrons between the atoms. It is this characteristic that enables water to act as a broad spectrum solvent. When a salt, such as silver nitrate, is added to water, it is able to dissolve, or dissociate its oppositely charged components. These charged components are suspended among the water molecules because of the electrostatic attraction between the charged components of the salt and the charged water molecules. The conventional use of the word "ionic" refers to this kind of relationship.

In the cathodic method of making colloidal silver, silver particles are "sintered" or broken off of the positive silver electrode and suspended in water. The separated silver particles can form in a variety of sizes ranging from single atoms to clusters consisting of a large number of atoms. A small particle that remains suspended in water is considered to be a colloid. In this discussion of ionic versus colloidal, some authorities regard a cluster of silver atoms carrying a positive charge to be an ion. The electrical attraction between a charged silver particle and the polar covalent water molecules is one of the factors that enables the silver colloidal particles to remain in suspension.

The differentiation between electrically charged microclusters of atoms and true ions can be difficult to determine. Many common methods for chemically testing silver content in water do not distinguish between colloidal and ionic forms. In these testing methods, acid is added to the liquid so that all of the colloidal particles are converted to ionic salts prior to testing. Electrical conductivity is affected by both ionic and colloidal forms of silver.

The Tyndall effect is an effect of light scattering by colloidal particles or particles in suspension. In a perfect ionic solution, one would expect the Tyndall effect to be absent. In a colloidal suspension, the Tyndall effect leaves a visible beam through the suspension.

Those authorities who believe that colloidal silver particles are more desirable than ionic silver generally agree that smaller particle size is desirable. Smaller particle sizes mean a greater surface area of silver per unit volume of silver and per unit weight of silver.

It is assumed that the cathodic process produces a combination of colloidal particles of various sizes and true ionic products. This would be a consequence of the electrolysis and impurities in the water and silver electrodes.

The simplest apparatus for generating silver colloids is a low voltage DC power source, a jar of distilled water, silver electrodes suspended in the water and a bit of wire to connect it all together. Any battery will work although a 6, 12, or 24 volt battery is ideal. One 9 volt transistor battery or two (18 VDC) or three (27 VDC) of them connected in series are also commonly used. The current drain is minimal and small batteries will last a long time. In Dr. Becker's research, they used 0.9 volts or less to diffuse silver directly into the tissues and fluids of a wound, and that was effective.

The cathodic method involves placing silver electrodes in a container of distilled water and passing a direct current through the water. A disruptive action takes place at the positive electrode resulting in fine particles of metallic silver being ripped away and suspended in the water. It is that simple.

While this basic technique is simple in principle, there are a few things that one must be careful about. Some batches made by this basic process turn out to be of relative high quality and stability and others may turn black and precipitate rather quickly.

Good quality distilled water has a very low electrical conductivity. In fact, absolutely pure water would be an electrical insulator. It is impurities in the water than enable it to conduct electricity. The more impurities present, the higher the electrical conductivity. Impurities may include dust particles, dissolved mineral salts and dissolved gases from the atmosphere. Too many impurities can produce unpredictable results because of the interaction of the impurities with the electrolytic process.

When silver electrodes are placed in the water and a DC voltage applied, the resulting current flow adds silver to the water. As silver enters the water, the electrical conductivity increases. Higher current densities increase the rate that silver is added to the water. It appears that higher current densities result in larger colloidal particle sizes as well as higher concentrations of silver suspended in the water. When a constant voltage source is used, this process becomes self limiting because increasing particle size leads to conglomeration of small silver particles into larger ones and precipitation of larger particles. The electrical charge between the two electrodes suspended in the water can act as a kind of electrostatic precipitator. This puts an upper limit on the concentration of silver that can be suspended in water to about 20 parts per million, depending on some process variables. Other techniques can produce higher concentrations.

The manufacturing process can be dramatically improved by replacing the constant voltage source with a constant current source. A constant current source limits the current density of the current flowing between the silver electrodes. This, in turn, reduces the production of larger, potentially unstable silver particles.

There are a number of companies and individuals who have built and marketed constant current silver generators or plans on how to make them. One of these companies is Silvergen (www.silvergen.com).

Trem Williams, founder of Silvergen, offered this information. Two key factors in producing stable high quality colloidal silver are:

- Maintain the current density in a window between 1 and 2 milliamperes per square inch of electrode surface.

- Stir or circulate the liquid while the current is flowing.

While the electronic variables in the production process can be precisely controlled, the quality of the distilled water is much more difficult to control. Distilled water (not bottled drinking water) from the grocery store is usually satisfactory, but not always. Distilled water made in a home distiller was a dismal failure. It contained far too many contaminants. Manufacturers who are determined to produce a superior product use laboratory grade deionized water.

Some of the colloidal silver making kits on the market recommend adding a pinch of sea salt to the water to increase conductivity. Those doing this should be aware that an electrochemical reaction will occur between the silver and the chlorine ions forming silver chloride. The silver chloride may form as colloidal silver chloride particles rather than silver colloids. Silver chloride is slightly soluble in water so some silver ions would also be present. Silver chloride is not the same product as colloidal silver.

The reason some people add salt to the water is to increase conductivity. Current flow is necessary to break away the silver microclusters from the electrodes. Supermarket grade distilled water has enough impurities to allow it to conduct enough current to get the process started. If you use laboratory grade distilled water, you can use very high voltages or high voltage arcs to get the process to work. Another alternative is to add a small amount of colloidal silver from a previous batch to the distilled water to make it minimally conductive and get the process started. You can then continue using the low voltage DC setup.

Any inorganic impurities in the water will also participate in the electrochemical reaction and produce a variety of silver salts, some likely soluble and some likely insoluble. The presence of unknown compounds adds uncertainty about the quality and stability of the product. The presence of "any" organic matter may provoke precipitation of the colloidal silver.

The containers and other materials should be cleaned very thoroughly before use with distilled water only. Many soap and detergent residues can spoil a batch of colloidal silver. It would be wise to clean the container and electrodes with distilled water before running a trial batch. In some situations, the process can be sensitive to the contaminants in the glass and plastic of the containers themselves.

I have had good results with glass containers and food grade polyethylene 5 gallon buckets for both making and storing colloidal silver. Silicone (used as a sealant around plumbing connectors), even though it was food grade, caused precipitation on prolonged contact.

The electrodes should be made of pure silver. You can contact a local mint or a mint in a nearby city and obtain .9995 fine silver in a variety of forms. (The .05% impurity is mostly copper.) For electrodes, the stock used to stamp out silver medallions is a good configuration and it can be cut to length. Sometimes you can get raw material through a jeweler. For very small setups, some companies sell high purity silver wlre. .999 fine silver rounds can be used for small batches. Jewelry, silverware, and old silver coins won't give a pure product because they are not pure silver. They should be avoided.

The silver electrodes themselves can become contaminated either with mineral contaminants picked up from the water, organic contaminants, or products of the surface chemistry of the electrodes. If this occurs, the production of stable silver colloids can become impaired and you have to either change the electrodes or thoroughly clean them. During the electrolytic process a black coating will form on the negative - pole and a golden gray slimy mass may form on the positive + pole. This is not a problem. The black material is silver oxide and the gray slimy stuff is precipitated silver particles.

High voltages, both DC and AC have been used to form electrical arcs between the silver electrodes and the water surface. For safety and simplicity, it is probably best to stick to low voltage DC methods unless you are sufficiently technically adept to handle potentially lethal currents and voltages safely, or if you can afford one of the commercial HVAC units.

As the water accumulates silver, the color can range from clear to yellow or golden. The color is a function of particle size. The small particles will produce a clear or nearly clear liquid which will also display a Tyndall effect. Larger particles will be light yellow. As the particles get larger, the color will become a darker yellow or golden, then red, then green and finally blue. The largest particles produce a blue color.

When the process is stopped, you need to filter the liquid into a clean container. One choice of filter is the Katadyn ceramic cartridge filter. This filter will remove any particles, including bacteria cells, larger than 0.2 microns. You can get the hand pump versions that are carried by backpackers or a larger under the sink model to which you have to add a pump. These filter elements can be cleaned when they clog up. Even though these filters have very small pores, the colloidal particles which are on the order of .001 to .01 microns in size pass through with ease.

You need to be aware of the stability limitations of colloidal silver. A colloid consists of very small particles suspended in water. The colloidal particles are subject to precipitation over time. True ionic solutions may have a photochemical reaction to light, while colloidal particles of silver do not. The two factors which affect the stability of good quality colloidal silver are exposure to contaminants and exposure to electric and magnetic fields.

In my experiments, I had samples that sat on a shelf for over a decade with no precipitation. I also observed that heat, cold, and light exposure had no effect on the silver suspension. The one factor which colloidal silver suspensions are very sensitive to is exposure to electric and magnetic fields. This includes the electrostatic fields often carried on the bodies and clothing of people. Samples sitting near walkways with moving people became unstable and precipitated, while samples from the same batch, using the same type of containers, that were separated by distance remained stable.

Some manufacturers add a protein or polymer to the suspension to stabilize it and prevent precipitation. Silver binds readily to proteins and if you add a stabilizing colloidal protein, like gelatin, you can prevent the precipitation of the silver. Many protein stabilized colloidal silver preparations should not be administered by injection because the protein may add to the toxicity. There are exceptions but they have to be carefully chosen.

Government Regulation of Colloidal Silver

On August 17, 1999, the FDA "finalized" its ruling against all OTC (over the counter) drugs containing colloidal silver ingredients or silver salts, to become effective within 30 days, as of September 16, 1999. The FDA "final rule" can be read in its entirety in the federal register. The document can be accessed at:

http://www.fda.gov/OHRMS/DOCKETS/98fr/081799a.pdf#xml=http://www.verity.fda.gov/search97cgi/s97_cgi.exe?action=View&VdkVgwKey=http%3A%2F%2Fwww%2Efda%2Egov%2FOHRMS%2FDOCKETS%2F98fr%2F081799a%2Epdf&doctype=xml&Collection=all&QueryZip=colloidal+silver&hlnavigate=ALL

The summary is that all silver products are classified as unapproved OTC drugs if any labeling statements are made that suggests that the products have any therapeutic benefits or can be used to treat any health condition. Now that the formality of posting announcements in the federal register and receiving responses has been fulfilled, the FDA is in a position to engage in enforcement actions against those who are not in compliance. Silver products can still be sold as nutritional products as long as they meet all regulations applicable to nutritional supplements and absolutely no medical claims are made about them.

Prior to this process, someone had requested and received from the FDA a letter indicating that colloidal silver could be marketed and sold as an OTC drug rather than a "new drug" provided that it had been manufactured and labeled exactly as it had been prior to 1938. This was an application of the "grandfather clause" allowing drugs marketed prior to the existence of the FDA to continue being marketed without having to go through the new drug application and approval process. This letter was rescinded shortly thereafter but marketers continued to publish claims of "FDA approval" long afterward. To be qualified as a grandfathered item, a product has to be in continuous production, manufactured in exactly the pre-1938 process, and labeled exactly in the pre-1938 manner. Colloidal Silver was not being made in the pre-1938 methods, it had not been in continuous production, and the labeling didn't match pre-1938 labels either. In light of what we know today, some of the pre-1938 products, their uses and misuses, and the advertising that went with them were toxic and hazardous.

Caught in the middle of this mess were a few physicians, ethical manufacturers, curious researchers, and sincere individuals who were in no way dishonest.

More recently, several companies have had process and application patents for manufacturing and using colloidal silver approved. Having a patent awarded does not, however, convey FDA approval. Given the flurry of new patents very recently, it is clear that the anti microbial properties of silver as caught the attention of researchers and business people who can see the potential for developing new products.

The FDA has issued approval for several silver products for topical application. These include silver dressings and bandages for topical use. Silvadene (Silver Sulfadiazine) cream made by Marion Laboratories is FDA approved as an antifungal and antibacterial cream for external use. It requires a prescription.

AgION is an antimicrobial powder coating. AgION is registered with the EPA, and with the FDA for use as an additive in food contact polymers. The National Sanitation Foundation has certified AgION as safe and acceptable for product zone and food zone applications.

Even more recently, a new regulatory effort has been introduced. The Environmental Protection Agency, EPA, is preparing to classify colloidal silver as a pesticide. No, silver does not kill insects. The argument is that silver discharged into the waste water from colloidal silver use and the discharge from silver containing washing machines and clothing, etc. *might* kill beneficial microorganisms.

Do silver discharges represent a risk to the ecosystem? That is a fair question, but it appears there is no proof that it does. So, the proposal is to require manufacturers to prove that it doesn't adversely affect the ecosystem. I don't recall the same restrictions ever being applied to chemical plants, oil refineries, *real* pesticide plants, and a host of other environmental hazards. Some individuals suspect that this is a ploy to eliminate small producers of silver products so large companies can claim the territory. As this is being written, the EPA is still taking comments on this issue. (113)(114)(115)

The Future of Colloidal Silver

So what is the future of colloidal silver?

The recent flurry of new silver product patents suggests that colloidal silver and related silver products are going to lose their orphan status.

As silver and silver products are recognized as safe and effective, the market potential is enormous. The question then is, "Who will profit by supplying that market?"

Appendix A - List of pre and post 1938 Documented Uses for Colloidal Silver

H.E.L.P.ful NEWS (36) published a summary of the various diseases, general conditions, and disease organisms whose successful treatment with colloidal silver was reported in both pre and post 1938 publications. These different sources used different formulations and concentrations of colloidal silver and were not always very specific about their treatment protocols. They have in common that they were claiming success in using some form of silver as a therapeutic agent. The following summary is quoted from their publication (36):

Please note that the spelling is quoted directly from the references of the period. This is usually from the early 1900's and many of the references were British using British spelling conventions.

"The following is a collection of conditions and pathogens we have found documented before 1938 where patients were being successfully treated using colloidal silver:"

"Anthrax Bacilli (12), (13)
Appendicitis (13)
Axillae and Blind Boils of the Neck (10)
B. Coli (12)
B. Coli Communis (17)
B. Dysentery (14)
B. Tuberculosis (17)
Bacillary Dysentery (14)
Bladder Irritation (22)
Blepharitis (23)
Boils (20)
Bromidrosis in Axille (22)
Bromidrosis in Feet (20)
Burns and Wounds of the Cornea (23)
Cerebrospinal Meningitis (13), (19)
Chronic Cystitis (20)
Chronic Eczema of Anterior Nares (20)
Chronic Eczema of Maetus of Ear (20)
Colitis (14)

Cystitis (12)
Dacrycystitis (23)
Dermatitis suggestive of Toxaemia (14)
Diarrhoea (14)
Diphtheria (13)
Dysentery (13), (16)
Ear Affections (13)
Enlarged Prostate (22)
Epididymitis (20)
Erysipelas (13)
Eustachian Tubes (patency restored) (12)
Follicular Tonsillitis (20)
Furunculosis (13)
Gonococcus (17)
Gonorrhea (20)
Gonorrheal Conjunctivitis (20)
Gonorrheal Opthalimia (23)
Gonorrheal Prostatic Gleet (21)
Hemorrhoids (22)
Hypophyon Ulcer (23)
Impetigo (20)
Infantile Disease (26)
Infected Ulcers of the Cornea (23)
Inflammatory Rheumatism (13)
Influenza (21)
Intestinal Keratitis (23)
Intestinal Troubles (16)
Lesion Healing (22)
Leucorrhoea (16)
Menier's Syndrome (16)
Nasal Catarrh (15)
Nasopharyngeal Catarrh (reduced) (18)
Oedematous enlargement of Turbinates without True Hyperplasia (20)
Offensive Discharge of Chronic Suppuration in Otitis Media (20)
Ophthalmology (12)
Ophthalmic practices (13)
Para-Typhoid (13)
Paramecium (11)
Perineal Eczema (22)
Phelgmons (13)
Phlyctenular Conjunctivitis (20)
Pneumococci (12)
Pruritis Ani (22)
Puerperal Septicemia (25)
Purulent Opthalmia of Infants (23)

Pustular Eczema of Scalp (20)
Pyorrhoea Alveolaris (Riggs Disease) (18)
Quinsies (16)
Rhinitis (19)
Ringworm of the body (20)
Scarlatina (13)
Sepsis (26)
Septic Tonsillitis (20)
Septic Ulcers of the legs (20)
Septicaemia (15), (18)
Shingles (16)
Soft Sores (20)
Spring Catarrh (20)
Sprue (16)
Staphyloclysin (inhibits) (12)
Staphylococcus Pyogenea (17)
Staphylococcus Pyogens Albus (12)
Staphylococcus Pyogens Aureus (12)
Streptococci (17)
Subdues Inflammation (22)
Suppurative Appendicitis (post-op) (20)
Tinea Versicolor (20)
Tonsillitis (16)
Typhoid (13)
Typhoid Bacillus (24)
Ulcerative Urticaria (14)
Urticaria suggestive of Toxaemia (22)
Valsava's Inflammation (16)
Vincent's Angina (20)
Vorticella (11)
Warts (22)
Whooping cough (16)"

One has to also remember that medical journals and books from this period often tended to use and promote a wide variety of treatments as universal cures for most everyhing. Some ingenious and effective therapies were pushed out of use by the medical economic system and others were abandoned because they were so atrocious that they never should have been used at all. The fact that silver products were the standard in treating infections for decades is one indication that they should be reconsidered using modern scientific knowledge and tools. Just because it is old does not mean that it is not valid.

The same article lists the following uses from post 1938 sources.

"Adenovirus 5 (33)
Asper Gillus Niger (28)
Bacillus Typhosus (31)
Bovine Rotavirus (33)
Candida Albicans (28)
Endamoeba Histolytica (cysts) (34)
Escherichia Coli (27), (28), (21)
Legionella Pneumophila (27)
Poliovirus 1 (Sabin Strain) (33)
Pseudomonas Aeruginosa (27), (28)
Salmonella (32)
Spore-Forming Bacteria (31)
Staphylococcus Aureus (27)
Streptococcus Faecalis (27)
Vegetative B. Cereus Cells (34)"

The same article lists the following as a documented list of silver resistant bacteria.

"Citrobacter Freundii (30)
Enterobacter Cloacae (30)
Enterobacteriaceae (some strains) (29)
Escherichia Coli (some strains) (29)
Klebsiella Pneumoniae (30)
P. Stutzeri (some strains) (29)
Proteus Mirabilis (30)
Vegetative B. Cereus Spores (34)"

Appendix B – List of Pathogens Killed by American Silver Products

US Patent No 7135195 was issued to American Silver, LLC on November 14, 2006. This company claims that their product is 97% metallic silver colloids with essentially no ions present. The following list from the patent shows the actual concentration of their colloidal silver solution required to kill specific pathogens. This information is listed for reference and comparison purposes because it shows that silver colloids are highly germicidal against these common pathogens. You will note the concentrations are very low, the highest being just 10 parts (of silver) per million (PPM):

At 5.0 ppm Staphylococcus aureus was killed
At 5.0 ppm Osteomyelitis Staphylococcus aureus was killed
At 2.5 ppm Bacillary Dysentery Shigella boydii was killed
At 5.0 ppm Burn Infections Pseudomonas aeruginosa was killed
At 5.0 ppm Dental Plaque Streptococcus mutans was killed
At 2.5 ppm Diarrhea (Bloody) Shigella boydii was killed
At 2.5 ppm Diarrhea Escherichia coli was killed
At 1.25 ppm Ear Infection Haemophilus influenzae was killed
At 2.5 ppm Ear Infection Streptococcus pneumonie was killed
At 2.5 ppm Enteric Fever Salmonella tyhimurium was killed
At 1.25 ppm Epiglottitis (In children) Haemophilus influenzae killed
At 5.0 ppm Eye Infections Staphylococcus aureus was killed
At 5.0 ppm Corneal Ulcers-Keratitis Pseudomonas aeruginosa killed
At 5.0 ppm Food Poisoning Salmonella arizona was killed
At 2.5 ppm Food Poisoning Salmonella tyhimurium was killed
At 2.5 ppm Food Poisoning Escherichia coli was killed
At 2.5 ppm Endocarditis Streptococcus faecalis was killed
At 5.0 ppm Endocarditis Streptococcus gordonii was killed
At 1.25 ppm Meningitis Haemophilus influenzae was killed
At 2.5 ppm Meningitis Enterobacter aerogenes was killed
At 5.0 ppm Meningitis Pseudomonas aeruginosa was killed
At 2.5 ppm Meningitis Streptococcus pneumonie was killed
At 2.5 ppm Nosocomial Infections Klebsiella pneumoniae was killed
At 5.0 ppm Nosocomial Infections Pseudomonas aeruginosa killed
At 1.25 ppm Nosocomial Infections (From Strep.pyogenes) killed
At 5.0 ppm Pneumonia Staphylococcus aureus was killed
At 1.25 ppm Pneumonia Haemophilus influenzae was killed
At 5.0 ppm Pneumonia Pseudomonas aeruginosa was killed
At 2.5 ppm Pneumonia Streptococcus pneumonie was killed
At 1.25 ppm Respiratory Tract Infections Strep. pyogenes was killed

At 2.5 ppm Respiratory Tract Infections E. coli was killed
At 2.5 ppm Respiratory Tract Infections Klebsiella pneumoniae killed
At 1.25 ppm Scarlet Fever Streptococcus pyogenes was killed
At 2.5 ppm Septicemia Enterobacter aerpyogenes was killed
At 1.25 ppm Sinus Infections Haemophilus influenzae was killed
At 2.5 ppm Sinusitis Streptococcus pneumonie was killed
At 1.25 ppm Impetigo Staphylococcus aureus was killed
At 5.0 ppm Skin Infections Staphylococcus aureus was killed
At 1.25 ppm Skin Infections Streptococcus pyogenes was killed
At 1.25 ppm Strep Throat Streptococcus pyogenes was killed
At 1.25 ppm Suppurative Arthritis Haemophilus influenzae killed
At 1.25 ppm Throat Infections Haemophilus influenzae was killed
At 5.0 ppm Tooth Decay Streptococcus mutans was killed
At 10.0 ppm Urethritis (Men) Trichomonas vaginalis was killed
At 2.5 ppm Urinary Tract Infections E. coli was killed
At 2.5 ppm Urinary Tract Infections Klebsiella pneumoniae killed
At 5.0 ppm Urinary Tract Infections Pseudomonas aeruginosa killed
At 2.5 ppm Urinary Tract Infections Streptococcus faecalis killed
At 2.5 ppm Urinary Tract Infections Enterobacter aerpyogenes killed
At 10.0 ppm Vaginitis (Women) Trichomonas vaginalis was killed
At 2.5 ppm Wound Infections Escherichia coli was killed
At 2.5 ppm Wound Infections Enterobacter aerpyogenes was killed
At 2.5 ppm Wound Infections Klebsiella pneumoniae was killed
At 5.0 ppm Wound Infections Pseudomonas aeruginosa was killed
At 2.5 ppm Wound Infections Streptococcus faecalis was killed
At 10.0 ppm Yeast Infections Candida albicans was killed

Appendix C - Correspondence and Reports from Colloidal Silver Users

The following summaries are a few examples of reports and communications from individuals who have used colloidal silver.

In 2000, I posted a request for information on personal use of colloidal silver and the results obtained. This request was made to the silver list.

Illness, Disease, or symptoms present at time of treatment? *A 64 year old man with history normal childhood diseases: mumps, measles, whooping cough. Have had smallpox vax. Hepatitis A or B at age 32. Heavy alcohol use prior to Hep. Lingering liver pain following 3 year recovery from Hep. No longer any dull liver ache following several years of CS. Infection in right tibia from scratch on anterior shin led to multiple courses of Keflex for cellulitus. Followed by pitting edema of shin for years. Kroger Herbs "Circuflow" reduced swelling. Tinea Pedis all adult life. Small blisters and flaking and itching of skin. Tibia not normal with only rare and occasional swelling apparently connected with sitting too long. Dental health better: fewer cavities; gums never infected. Toenail fungus improved, but not eliminated. Some type of warts immediately removed. "Flat Warts" highly resistant as they shrink to about 2 mm.*

Professional Diagnosis? (yes/no): *Yes.*

Response of symptoms to treatment? *In 1996 I began making CS using 3 9Vbatts with 14 gauge Ag .999 fine hanging in glass. Salt used at 1/2 amount specified by Metcalf process [Silversolutins device]. Athlete's foot gone in 3 months. No topical use. With use of CsPro HVAC machine for about 3 years, Liver pain gone. Gum infections now do not occur. Consumption is about 2 oz per day, not consistent. Had Herpes Simples all adult life.*
Lesion on lip about 2 X annually. After three months of HVAC CS, have not had recurrence for several years. Male friend with genital herpes has had same experience. Have had 1 mild flu in 3 years; others were sick weeks; I was sick 3 days.

That treated with the LVDC CS. In 3 Years: 1 cold, mild, and 1 Upper respiratory minor 1 day cough and strange whitephlegm. Some said it was chemtrails. Excellent results treating burns and cuts. Effects on burns is astounding; no infection, rapid healing; almost invisible scarring.

Side Effects Noted of Suspected? *None*

Brand or Source of CS? *Self Made. CSPro Ultra Professional. Nominal 10KV 60 Hz. Submerged electrode plate on one side of secondary, with suspended wires on other side of secondary; just above water surface which draw cones up about 3/8 inch.*

Concentration (PPM)? *Varies from about 8 to over 10. Difficulty making higher concentrations. I have a spectrophotometer and test mg/L with Hach reagents.*

Dosage? *I never really kept track due to the low toxicity of Ag colloid. Probably 8 oz a day when I had the flu, using the LVDC CS. Now, I take a sip most every day. Probably one to two ounces per day. US Fluid Ounces.*

Frequency of Dosage? *Almost every day.*

Duration of Treatment? *About 4 years.*

Total volume of CS consumed? *I don't know.*

Total Milligrams of CS consumed? *I don't know.*

Use Prophylacticaly? (yes/no): *Yes*

Prophylactic Dosage? *See above*

How Long? *About 4 years.*

Illness, Disease, or symptoms present at time of treatment? *sinus/chest cold + ear infection.*

Professional Diagnosis? (yes/no): *No*

Response of symptoms to treatment? *100% within 4 hrs. for ears, ~90% relief within 10 hrs. for chest/throat, 75% relief within 72 hrs for sinus.*

Side Effects Noted of Suspected? *None*

Brand or Source of CS? *HVAC home brew.*

Concentration (PPM)? *Made 26 PPM, diluted to 10.7 PPM for storage & 1 PPM used.*

Dosage? *Dropper for ears, ~ 5 cc. spray down throat for lung & throat congestion & sprayed 2-3 cc. in nose (head upside down) for sinus infection.*

Frequency of Dosage? *Ears:1X, throat:~10X in 24 hrs., sinus: 2X in 24 hrs.*

Duration of Treatment? *10 sec.*

Total volume of CS consumed? *~ 50 cc in 24 hrs.*

Total Milligrams of CS consumed? *0.05 mg.*

Use Prophylacticaly? (yes/no): *Yes to brush teeth after normal brushing.*

Prophylactic Dosage? *1 cc*

How Long? *6 months*

Illness, Disease, or symptoms present at time of treatment? *Toenail fungus, various wounds*

Professional Diagnosis? (yes/no): *No*

Response of symptoms to treatment? *Treatment unintentional byproduct of making and tasting CS. Fungus*

90% gone in two years. Wounds heal right up with no scarring. [busted mechanics knuckles in only 2 days instead of many] One sore throat in 3 yrs that didn't last more than 2 hrs accompanied by that "beat with a pipe" feeling for 1 1/2 days...but never got really ill. Zero cavities or plaque from the date of starting CS [very unusual for me] Continual 15+ yr battle with ringworm is almost forgotten.

Side Effects Noted of Suspected? *None*

Brand or Source of CS? *Coyote Zenterprizes*

Concentration (PPM)? *Average 12 PPM*

Dosage? *A swallow and [later in the year] a soaking of the socks in the morning when worn. Frequency of Dosage: 2x per day.*

Duration of Treatment? *2 years*

Total volume of CS consumed? *5 gallons?*

Total Milligrams of CS consumed? *???*

Use Prophylacticaly? (yes/no): *Yes*

Illness, Disease, or symptoms present at time of treatment? *Medically diagnosed by conventional means, with supporting labs or testing processes:*

(1) Raynauds disease (severe)
(2) Chronic Fatigue Syndrome
(3) Prolapsed mitral valve with regurgitation
(4) Congestive heart failure (2 occasions)
(5) Neurally mediated hypotension
(6) Ringing in the ears
(7) Vascular accidents (several - diagnosed by MRI) frontal lobe and both sides.

(8) ITP (idiopathic Thromboletic Purpura) or a blood clotting problem which results in a rash like over trunk, upper arms, etc.
(9) Chronically low blood pressure and pulse.
(10) Trouble maintaining adequate weight (have to work hard to maintain a safe weight limit, and not lose too much weight. Am now only slightly thin (small build anyway).

Professional Diagnosis? (yes): *And documented by conventional means.*

Response of symptoms to treatment? *Well, I am still alive and breathing, although energy, concentration, and health are not the greatest.*

Side Effects Noted of Suspected? *Not sure.*

Brand or Source of CS? *Have a small CS generator, and make it at home. Unsure of the concentration, or ppm, as I have only been doing this for a month, and have no equipment other than the cheap little CS generator. Am still learning as I go. The CS has a slight yellow color, and has been consistent in taste and color.*

Concentration (PPM)? *Unknown*

Dosage? *4 ounces daily, two AM and two PM.*

Frequency of Dosage? *Two ounces AM, and two PM.*

Duration of Treatment? *Treatment has been for approximately 3 weeks now. Total volume of CS consumed: 4 ounces daily.*

Total Milligrams of CS consumed? *4 ounces daily*

Use Prophylacticaly? (yes): *After remission of the chronic fatigue syndrome, I will continue to use CS on a regular basis. I will use CS and alternate, following the protocol used for doxycycline treatment for CFS, which is 6 weeks on and one week off, and then repeat, until symptoms resolve. I will continue this process for at least two years.*

Prophylactic Dosage? *Not applicable at this point.*

Illness, Disease, or symptoms present at time of treatment? *Chronic extreme sinusitis, general lethargy.*

Professional Diagnosis? (yes/no): *Yes, no (to above)*

Response of symptoms to treatment? *Some apparent help, big increase in energy.*

Side Effects Noted of Suspected? *None*

Brand or Source of CS? *Homemade*

Concentration? (PPM): *About 12*

Dosage? *2 oz*

Frequency of Dosage? *4-8 times daily*

Duration of Treatment? *?? been drinking it for 3+ years (initially 1 oz daily).*
Total volume of CS consumed? *?*

Total Milligrams of CS consumed? *?*

Use Prophylacticaly ? (yes/no): *Yes*

Prophylactic Dosage? *Varies*

I tested various uses for CS prior to using it on myself. I first used it externally on plants and pets, to see what effects it had. Then tried it as an external disinfectant/aid for bites, acne, athlete's foot, ingrown toenail, etc. Only then did I try it internally -- first in pets' water, then mine (and my sons') and as a nasal spray and eye drops. So far, no negative side effects in any trial -- only neutral or positive.

From Trem Williams, (www.silvergen.com)

Our vet has a horse which had an abscessed tendon on its fetlock which was swollen and continually draining. It also had a continuous fever. She was unable to affect a cure using antibiotics. She took it to a veterinary hospital where it received surgery and stayed for about six weeks. They were unable to help the horse and told her it would be a limping pasture horse at best if it lived. They said it would probably never be able to carry anyone again. She brought it home and it continued to hobble and stand around.

She (the vet) came to work on our horse and she happened to mention the story I just described. She was quite sad about the state of the horse.

I offered her some of our 15 PPM CS (2 liters) and she said she would try it as a last resort since nothing else had worked.

Using a syringe without needle, she irrigated the wound with CS. She also gave it several ounces orally and went to bed.

Upon rising, she noticed the horse was frolicking in its corral. She went to investigate and noticed the wound had stopped draining for the first time in many weeks. The swelling was greatly reduced overnight. The fever had also disappeared. She continued to give 4 ounces of CS orally daily until the CS was gone. I believe she irrigated the wound 1 or 2 more times in the next day or so.

The fever never returned. The wound completely healed and the horse is now being ridden by her children. Total recovery. No placebo affect there!

From a reader:

My daughter has a cat that was very ill. Her cat was acting delirious, was unable to stand, and she was concerned that the animal was dying. She gave it a small quantity of colloidal silver and within 24 hours, it was acting normally, eating and playing like a kitten. I know a family who raises exotic breeds of cats and crosses with wild breeds. These cats, when raised in captivity, tend to be susceptible to many common infections, especially of the eyes and respiratory tract. They give their animals very small amounts of colloidal silver in their drinking water and use it topically when they get ill and tell glowing stories of cures of eye, oral and respiratory infections. It is questionable whether enough silver being is delivered to have a significant germicidal effect.

From a reader:

I work in a silver mint. We were recovering silver from silver chloride tablets salvaged from military surplus survival kits (they used it to precipitate salt out of seawater to make it more or less potable) and I inhaled a lot of silver chloride dust from the air. That night I got very ill and the next day went to the doctor. I told them what I had been doing and they promptly ran a blood test and freaked out. They gave me a transfusion to reduce the excess silver levels. After that I felt fine, had no after effects and haven't had a single cold, flu, or any other illness in the fifteen years following that incident.

The following exchange took place by e-mail with an individual who wishes to remain anonymous:

"I was on argyrol when a child. My skin is pigmented now and I understand there is no known cure on how to change the pigmentation. Sure wish something could be done. Let me be the first to know."

>Thank you for your comments. Regrettably, I have found no reference in the medical literature for the removal of the silver pigmentation.

I am revising my colloidal silver document and request your permission to publish your comments in the correspondence section. Name deleted if you wish.

>I would also like to ask you a few questions:

>(1) What was being treated with the Argyrol?

"In reply to your above questions - yes you may publish my comments name deleted."

"As a child argyrol was administered to me in the form of nose drops. The treatment was for a sore throat. My mother thought this was a cure-all for everything so every time my brother or I sneezed here came the argyrol. "

>(2) Was the treatment effective?

" But, I have to admit the treatment was effective. "

>(3) How much did you take and over what period of time?

"I'm going to guess the approximate length of time we used argyrol was maybe 6 mos. to a year when the Doctor finally looked at us and asked my mom to STOP administering argyrol immediately!!"

>(4) Some people believe that having silver stored in their organs and tissues confers resistance to infections. Do you see any evidence that this may or may not be true?

"I consider myself very lucky as I seldom get infections - maybe the flu once a year, but that's probably because I want a day off work!"

From a reader:

"My son had the mumps with the usual fever, malaise and swelling. We gave him a large dose of colloidal silver and within 24 hours all his symptoms were gone." (Note: the dose in this case was a 32 oz. bottle of 1 PPM colloidal silver)

The following summary is summarized from the Orem Herald, Feb. 13, 1992.

Darkly Tichy, a member of the administrative staff at the Brigham Young University, engaged in private research on colloidal silver. He had his electrically produced colloidal silver tested at several labs and determined that the silver killed a variety of pathogens including HIV virus. He injected in into his 6 year old son who had about 70 warts on his hands. He claimed that all the warts cleared up after one injection. Tichy lacked the credentials and financial support to gain mainstream acceptance of his colloidal silver by organized medicine and the FDA. "It's like saying, 'Here is the answer that everyone is looking for, but no one wants to find.'"

From a reader:

I had a rash from causes unknown. I sprayed colloidal silver on it. After two applications, it was gone

---

Appendix D – Recent Colloidal Silver Patents

This is a partial list of some recent patents regarding colloidal silver, silver products and their applications in treating human diseases. This is not a comprehensive list.

US Patent No. 7,435,438, Arata, October 14, 2008.

Disinfectant and method of use

A process is disclosed for treating consumable food products, the process comprising the step of applying to a consumable food product an aqueous disinfectant solution comprising silver dihydrogen citrate in an amount sufficient to obtain at least a 2.36 log.sub.10 reduction in the number of microorganisms present. Also disclosed is a process comprising applying to a consumable food product an aqueous disinfectant solution comprising from 5 PPM to 30 PPM of silver dihydrogen citrate and from 5% to 10% citric acid. Also disclosed is a process comprising exposing a consumable food product to from 5 PPM to 30 PPM of silver dihydrogen citrate for at least 5 seconds, allowing the food product to drip dry, and rinsing the food product with at least 0.1 PPM of silver dihydrogen citrate.

US Patent No. 7,445,799, Sarangapani, et al. November 4, 2008.

Compositions for microbial and chemical protection

An antimicrobial and chemical deactivating composition for use in a liquid medium or for incorporation into a coating, structural plastic materials, thin microporous membranes, textiles and sponges. The composition includes macrosize or submicron particles of silver, platinum with silver and their salts with parabens, oxide, salicylate, acetate, citrate, benzoate, and phosphate along with copper and zinc salts of the same.

US Patent No. 7,427,416, Gillis, et al. September 23, 2008.

Methods of treating conditions using metal-containing materials

Methods of treating conditions using metal-containing materials are disclosed. Exemplary conditions include bacterial conditions, biofilm conditions, microbial conditions, inflammatory conditions, fungal conditions, viral conditions, autoimmune conditions, idiopathic conditions, hyperproliferative conditions, noncancerous growths, cancerous conditions, and combinations of such conditions. In certain embodiments, the metal-containing material is an atomically disordered, nanocrystalline silver-containing material.

US Patent No. 7,457,667, Skiba, November 25, 2008.

Current producing surface for a wound dressing

In an embodiment, an article includes a primary surface and a pattern of spaced dissimilar materials, on the primary surface. The pattern is to spontaneously produce electrical surface currents when brought into contact with an electrically conducting solution. Dissimilar metals used to make the preferred embodiment of the present invention (a wound dressing) are silver and zinc, and the electrolytic solution includes sodium chloride in water. Bandages and wound dressings are simple, familiar devices. In an effort to hasten the wound healing process or reduce the risk of infection, there have been many recent efforts to redesign, or sometimes redefine, a bandage. Few people have enjoyed the benefits of some new bandages, because they are either too complex or too expensive.

US Patent No. 7,491,330, Harvey, February 17, 2009.

Silver chloride treated water purification device containing the porous grog and method for making same

A porous grog with a body composition of water, clay, and combustible material. Further, an earthenware water purification filter utilizing the porous grog in the body composition of the filter. Further, an earthenware filter utilizing silver chloride treatment for water disinfection is disclosed. A water purification system incorporating said filter, said water purification system capable of removing about 99% of all particles not less than 1.0 micron is size, and removing virtually 100% of fecal coliform indicators. In other embodiments, methods of disinfecting pottery toilet liners including various open surfaces using silver chloride treatment are disclosed.

US Patent No. 7,462,590, Tichy, et al. December 9, 2008.

Aqueous disinfectants and sterilants comprising a peroxide/peracid/transition metal mixture

The present invention is drawn to disinfectant or sterilant compositions and associated methods of use. In one embodiment, an aqueous disinfectant or sterilant composition can comprise an aqueous vehicle, including water, from 0.001 wt % to 50 wt % of a peracid, and from 0.001 wt % to 25 wt % of a peroxide. Additionally, from 0.001 PPM to 50,000 PPM by weight of a transition metal based on the aqueous vehicle content can also be present. The disinfectant composition can be used in the manufacture of disinfectant wipes, disinfectant gels, and disinfectant fogs. In one embodiment, the composition can be substantially free of aldehydes. Alternatively or additionally, the transition metal can be in the form of a colloidal transition metal.

US Patent No. 7,455,851, Nelson, et al. November 25, 2008.

Pyrithione biocides enhanced by silver, copper, or zinc ions

The present invention is directed to an antimicrobial composition, comprising pyrithione or a pyrithione complex; and a zinc or copper or silver source selected from the group consisting of zinc or copper or silver salts, oxides, hydroxides, sulfates, chlorides, metals, and combinations thereof; wherein the weight ratio of the zinc or copper or silver source to the pyrithione or the pyrithione complex is in the range from about 1:300 to about 50:1, and wherein the antimicrobial composition has an enhanced biocidal effect against a variety of free-living microorganisms or biofilms. Also disclosed is a method of inhibiting the growth of free-living microorganisms or biofilm utilizing the above antimicrobial composition, as well as use of such antimicrobial compositions in various products including fuels, fluids, lubricants, coatings, adhesives, sealants, elastomers, soaps, cosmetics, plastic or woven or non-woven fibers, pharmaceuticals, and as preservatives for the above products.

US Patent No. 7,402,239, Dorward, July 22, 2008.

Water purification apparatus and method of using the same

A water purification apparatus, comprising a water pump, wherein the water pump inlet port receives water from an external source, a nonreturn valve in fluid communication with the water pump outlet port, and an ionizer chamber in fluid communication with the nonreturn valve output end, wherein the ionizer chamber doses a bacteriacide into water contained in the ionizer chamber. The apparatus also includes a filter, wherein the input end of the filter is in fluid communication with the output end of the ionizer chamber. *Colloidal silver* is comprised of microscopic silver particles with a positive charge, i.e., Ag+ ions. In one embodiment, *colloidal silver* is pulled from a pure silver electrode immersed in contaminated water. The *colloidal silver* attaches to the contaminating particles to stabilize its charge, thus disabling the contamination and producing potable water. Drinking water containing *colloidal silver* is tasteless and odorless in small concentrations, and is not toxic to humans.

US Patent No. 7,378,156 Terry May 27, 2008

Antimicrobial compositions containing colloids of oligodynamic metals

The present invention relates to antimicrobial compositions, methods for the production of these compositions, and use of these compositions with medical devices, such as catheters, and implants. The compositions of the present invention advantageously provide varying release kinetics for the active ions in the compositions due to the different water solubilities of the ions, allowing antimicrobial release profiles to be tailored for a given application and providing for sustained antimicrobial activity over time. More particularly, the invention relates to polymer compositions containing colloids comprised of salts of one or more oligodynamic metal, such as silver. The process of the invention includes mixing a solution of one or more oligodynamic metal salts with a polymer solution or dispersion and precipitating a colloid of the salts by addition of other salts to the solution which react with some or all of the first metal salts. The compositions can be incorporated into articles or can be employed as a coating on articles such as medical devices. Coatings may be on all or part of a surface.

US Patent No. 7,351,684, Tichy, et al. April 1, 2008.

Aqueous disinfectants and sterilants including colloidal transition metals

The present invention is drawn to disinfectant or sterilant compositions, which are human safe, e.g., food grade or food safe. In one embodiment, an aqueous disinfectant or sterilant composition can comprise an aqueous vehicle, including water, from 0.001 wt % to 50 wt % of a peracid, and from 0.001 wt % to 25 wt % of a peroxide. Additionally, from 0.001 PPM to 50,000 PPM by weight of a transition metal based on the aqueous vehicle content can also be present. The composition can be formulated to include only food-grade ingredients. Alternatively or additionally, the transition metal can be in the form of a colloidal transition metal.

US Patent No. 7,329,301, Chang, et al. February 12, 2008.

Silver nanoparticles made in solvent

This invention relates to a composition of matter comprising associated predominantly silver nanoparticles, and a method of making the nanoparticles. It further relates to articles comprising the nanoparticles.

US Patent No. 7,311,927, Miner, et al. December 25, 2007.

Antiseptic solutions containing silver chelated with polypectate and EDTA

A liquid antiseptic and cleanser having improved long-term stability includes at least the following principal ingredients: deionized water, silver ion, polypectate, and ethylenediaminetetraaceticacid (EDTA). Presently preferred embodiments of the technology also include glycerine; 1,2-propanediol (a.k.a. propylene glycol); at least one surfactant from any of the families of alkylsulfates, sulfonates, alkanolamides, betaines, amine oxides, sarcosinates, and sulfosuccinates; and a buffering compound sufficient to achieve a pH value within a range of 7.2 to 7.8.

US Patent No. 7,261,905, Arata, et al. August 28, 2007.

Disinfectant and method of making

A non-toxic environmentally friendly aqueous disinfectant is disclosed for specific use as prevention against contamination by potentially pathogenic bacteria and virus. The aqueous disinfectant is formulated by electrolytically generating silver ions in water in combination with a citric acid. The aqueous disinfectant may include a suitable alcohol and/or a detergent. The aqueous disinfectant has been shown to be very effective at eliminating standard indicator organisms such as staphylococcus aureus, salmonella cholerasuis and pseudomonas aeruginosa.

US Patent No. 7,201,925, Gillis, April 10, 2007.

Treatment of ungual and subungual diseases

The treatment of ungual and subungual diseases is disclosed. A method for the treatment of an ungual or subungual disease of a subject, the method comprising: administering via a needleless injector an effective ungual or subungual disease treating amount of a metal-containing material to an area of the subject associated with said disease, wherein the metal-containing material is an atomically disordered, nanocrystalline material that contains a metal selected from the group consisting of silver, gold, platinum, and palladium.

US Patent No. 7,135,195, Holladay, et al. November 14, 2006.

<u>Treatment of humans with **_colloidal silver_** composition</u>

We disclose a colorless composition comprising silver particles and water, wherein said particles comprise an interior of elemental silver and an exterior of ionic silver oxide, wherein the silver particles are present in the water at a level of about 5 to 40 PPM, and wherein the composition manifests significant antimicrobial properties. Methods of use of the composition are described.

United States Patent Application _20030185889_ Kind Code A1 Yan, Jixiong; et al. October 2, 2003.

<u>Colloidal nanosilver solution and method for making the same</u>

The present invention provides a colloidal nanosilver solution which contains nanosilver particles having diameters between 1 nm and 100 nm. The silver content in the colloidal solution is between 0.001% to 0.4% by weight. The colloidal nanosilver solution also contains a gelling agent which includes, but is not limited to, starch or its derivative, cellulose or its derivative, polymer or copolymer of acrylate or acrylate derivative, polyvinyl pyrrolidone, alginic acid, and xanthogenated gel. The present invention also provides a method for making the colloidal nanosilver solution. The colloidal nanosilver solution prepared by this method does not contain any toxic or impure substances.

United States Patent Application *20020051823* Kind Code A1 Yan, Jixiong; et al. May 2, 2002.

Nanosilver-containing antibacterial and antifungal granules and methods for preparing and using the same

The present invention relates to nanosilver-containing antibacterial and antifungal granules ("NAGs"). The NAGs have longlasting inhibitory effect on a broad-spectrum of bacteria and fungi, which include, but are not limited to, Escherichia coli, Methicillin resistant Staphylococcus aureus, Chlamydia trachomatis, Providencia stuartii, Vibrio vulnificus, Pneumobacillus, Nitrate-negative bacillus, Staphylococcus aureus, Candida albicans, Bacillus cloacae, Bacillus allantoides, Morgan's bacillus (Salmonella morgani), Pseudomonas maltophila, Pseudomonas aeruginosa, Neisseria gonorrhoeae, Bacillus subtilis, Bacillus foecalis alkaligenes, Streptococcus hemolyticus B, Citrobacter, and Salmonella paratyphi C. The NAGs contain ground stalk marrow of the plant Juncus effuses L. which has been dispersed with nanosilver particles. The nanosilver particles are about 1-100 mn in diameter. Each of the nanosilver particles contain a metallic silver core which is surrounded by silver oxide. The present invention also provides a process for making the NAGs. The NAGs can be used in a variety of healthcare and industrial products. Examples of the healthcare products include, but are not limited to, ointments or lotions to treat skin trauma, soaking solutions or cleansing solutions for dental or women hygiene, medications for treating gastrointestinal bacteria infections, sexual related diseases, and eye diseases. Examples of industrial products include, but are not limited to, food preservatives, water disinfectants, paper disinfectants, construction filling materials (to prevent mold formation).

US Patent No. 6,939,568, Burrell, et al. September 6, 2005.

Treatment of inflammatory skin conditions

The invention relates to the use of one or more antimicrobial metals, most preferably silver, preferably formed with atomic disorder, and preferably in a nanocrystalline form, for the treatment of inflammatory skin conditions. The nanocrystalline antimicrobial metal of choice may be used in the form of a nanocrystalline coating of one or more antimicrobial metals, a nanocrystalline powder of one or more antimicrobial metals, or a solution containing dissolved species from a nanocrystalline powder or coating of one or more antimicrobial metals.

US Patent No. 6,890,953, Arata, May 10, 2005.

Process for treating water

A process is disclosed for treating impure water by introducing a solution of electrolyticially generated silver citrate into the impure water wherein the silver is electrolytically generated in a solution of citric acid and water.

US Patent No. 6,743,348, Holladay, et al. June 1, 2004.

Apparatus and method for producing antimicrobial silver solution

An apparatus and method for producing colloidal silver. A large-volume container, such as a fifteen gallon container, includes a hinged lid on which a rotational impeller is mounted along with several sets of electrodes that are electrically connected to a power transformer. The container is partially filled with water, and when the lid is closed, the sets of electrodes are disposed in communication with the water in a predetermined arrangement, and the impeller resides submerged in the water. Certain of the electrodes constitute silver wire. The power transformers convey current to the electrodes, preferably alternating current, at voltages sufficient to cause silver particles to separate from the silver wire and enter the solution in a stable, suspended state. The impeller is rotated, preferably continuously, to prevent the suspended silver from remaining in upper levels of the water, thereby dispersing the silver particles more uniformly throughout the volume of water.

US Patent No. 5,785,972, Tyler, July 28, 1998.

Colloidal silver, honey, and helichrysum oil antiseptic composition and method of application

A composition of matter comprising a therapeutically active compound with antiseptic and osmotic characteristics for treatment or therapy for burns and open wounds experienced by animals and man and in particular to the treatment of thermal burns on humans by use of spray, mist, dropper, or saturated bandage application of the solution disclosed. The compound in solution form composed of colloidal silver, helichrysum angustifolium or helichrysum italicum oil and raw honey emulsified with water soluble lecithin by agitation.

US Patent No. 7,179,849, Terry February 20, 2007.

Antimicrobial compositions containing colloids of oligodynamic metals

The present invention relates to antimicrobial compositions, methods for the production of these compositions, and use of these compositions with medical devices, such as catheters, and implants. The compositions of the present invention advantageously provide varying release kinetics for the active ions in the compositions due to the different water solubilities of the ions, allowing antimicrobial release profiles to be tailored for a given application and providing for sustained antimicrobial activity over time. More particularly, the invention relates to polymer compositions containing colloids comprised of salts of one or more oligodynamic metal, such as silver. The process of the invention includes mixing a solution of one or more oligodynamic metal salts with a polymer solution or dispersion and precipitating a colloid of the salts by addition of other salts to the solution which react with some or all of the first metal salts. The compositions can be incorporated into articles or can be employed as a coating on articles such as medical devices. Coatings may be on all or part of a surface.

US Patent No. 7,005,556, Becker, et al. February 28, 2006.

Multilayer wound dressing

A flexible, multilayer wound dressing with antibacterial and antifungal properties, together with methods for making the dressing. The dressing includes a layer of silver-containing fabric, a layer of absorbent material, and (optionally) a layer of a flexible air-permeable and/or water-impermeable material. The dressing can be used for prophylactic and therapeutic care and treatment of skin infections and surface wounds (including surgical incisions), as a packing material, and as a swab for surface cleaning.

US Patent No. 6,838,095, Newman, et al. January 4, 2005.

Ionic silver complex

The invention relates to a substantially non-colloidal solution made by combining ingredients comprising (a) water; (b) a source of free silver ions; and (c) a substantially non-toxic, substantially thiol-free, substantially water-soluble complexing agent.

US Patent No. 6,749,597, Frank, June 15, 2004.

Respiratory infection treatment device

A device and method for treating an illness or infection in the respiratory tract of a body is provided. The device administers an antimicrobial mist directly to the tissues to be treated, which coats the tissues in the respiratory tract where the infection is colonizing. The administration of the mist is reapplied in order to maintain a predetermined antimicrobial tissue density concentration of a uncompounded silver colloid suspended antimicrobial substance for a predetermined time period.

US Patent No. 5,676,977, Antelman, October 14, 1997.

Method of curing AIDS with tetrasilver tetroxide molecular crystal devices

The diamagnetic semiconducting molecular crystal tetrasilver tetroxide (Ag_4O_4) is utilized for destroying the AIDS virus, destroying AIDS synergistic pathogens and immunity suppressing moieties (ISM) in humans. A single intravenous injection of the devices is all that is required for efficacy at levels of about 40 PPM of human blood. The device molecular crystal contains two mono and two trivalent silver ions capable of "firing" electrons capable of electrocuting the AIDS virus, pathogens and ISM. When administered into the bloodstream, the device electrons will be triggered by pathogens, a proliferating virus and ISM, and when fired will simultaneously trigger a redox chelation mechanism resulting in divalent silver moieties which chelate and bind active sites of the entities destroying them. The devices are completely non-toxic. However, they put stress on the liver causing hepatomegaly, but there is no loss of liver function.

Appendix E - Colloidal Silver Internet Resources

The silver-list is a moderated forum for discussion of colloidal silver and related topics.

http://www.silverlist.org/

The following links offer additional information on Argyria.

http://rosemaryjacobs.com/

http://dermatology.cdlib.org/111/case_reports/argyria/wadhera.html

http://en.wikipedia.org/wiki/Argyria

http://www.argyria.info/

http://www.silvermedicine.org/argyria.html

http://emedicine.medscape.com/article/1069121-overview

http://dermnetnz.org/reactions/argyria.html

http://www.lef.org/protocols/prtcl-156.shtml

http://www.americanbiotechlabs.com/researchArticles/argyria.html

More links on the safety and toxicology aspects of silver.

http://www.silvergen.com/General/altman.pdf
Colloidal silver: Where does it go when You Drink it and How long does it stay there – Dr. Roger Altman (must read)

http://risk.lsd.ornl.gov/tox/profiles/silver_f_V1.shtml
-RAIS - Risk Assessment Toxicity Profile - Silver

http://www.atsdr.cdc.gov/toxprofiles/tp146-c2.pdf
Health Effects of Silver – Agency for Toxic Substances and Disease Registry

References

(1) ARGYRIA The Pharmacology of Silver, William R. Hill, M.D. & Donald M. Pillsbury, M.A., M.D., The Williams & Wilkins Company, 1939

(2) "Silver Compound aids in Bacterial Defense" American Metal Market, Feb. 10, 1995, V 103, n 28

(3) FDA Background statement on Colloidal Silver, Received Sept. 13, 1995

(4) "Silver - New Magic in Medicine", Science Digest, March 1978

(5) The Use of Colloids in Health and Disease, Albert B. Searle, Constable & Company LTD, London, 1919

(6) Ayurveda Life, Health and Longevity, Svoboda, Robert E., Penguin Books, 1992

(7) The Body Electric, Robert O. Becker, M.D., William Morrow, 1985

(8) From information published on the Internet (http://www.xpressnet.com/bhealthy) by Discovery Experimental and Development, Inc., a pharmaceutical company and Advantage Pharmaceuticals, 1825-A Main Street, Winnipeg, Manitoba, Canada R2V2A4, 800-877-5097

(9) Electrochemistry in Colloids and Dispersions, Edited by Raymond A. Mackay and John Texter, VCH Publishers, Inc., 1992, ISBN 1-56081-573-6

(10) News Group posting, misc.health.alternative, alt.folklore.herbs, alt.health.Ayurveda, by Leslie Taylor<raintree@bga.com>, 10/23/1995

(11) Bechhold, H. (1919), Colloids in biology and medicine, translated by J.G.M. Bullow. D. Van Nostrand Company: New York,

(12) Ibid. p. 368

(13) Ibid. p. 367

(14) Searle, A. B., (1919), The use of Colloids in Health and Disease, (Quoting from the British Medical Journal, May 12, 1917), E. P. Dutton & Company, New York) p. 82

(15) Ibid., (Quoting from the British Medical Journal, Jan. 15, 1917) p. 83

(16) Ibid., (Quoting Sir James Cantlie in the British Medical Journal, Nov. 15, 1913) p. 83

(17) Ibid., (Quoting Henry Crookes) p. 70

(18) Ibid., (Quoting J. Mark Hovell in the British Medical Journal, Dec. 15, 1917)
p. 86

(19) Ibid., (Quoting B. Seymour Jones) p. 86

(20) Ibid., (Quoting C.E.A. MacLeod in Lancet, Feb. 3, 1912) p. 83

(21) Ibid., (Quoting J. MacMunn in the British Medical Journal, 1917, I, 685) p. 86

(22) Ibid., (Quoting Sir Malcolm Morris in the British Medical Journal, May 12, 1917) p. 85

(23) Ibid., (Quoting A. Legge Roe in the British Medical Journal, Jan. 16, 1915)

(24) Ibid., (Quoting W.J. Simpson in Lancet, Dec. 12, 1914) pp. 71-72

(25) Ibid., (Quoting T.H. Anderson Wells in Lancet, Feb. 16, 1918) p. 85

(26) (1931) Index-Catalogue of the Library of the Surgeon General's Office United States Army, United States Printing Office, Washington, V. IX, p. 628

(27) Moyasar, T. Y., , Landeen, L. K., Messina, M. C., Kuta, S. M. Schulze, R., and Gerba, C. P. , (1990), Disinfection of Bacteria in Water Systems by using electrolytically generated copper:silver and reduced levels of free chlorine. Found in the Canadian Journal of Microbiology. The National Research Council of Canada: Ottawa, Ont. Canada. pp. 109-116

(28) Simonetti, N., Simonetti, G., Bougnol, F., and Scalzo, M. (1992) Electrochemical Ag+ for preservative use. Article found in Applied and Environmental Microbiology. American Society for Microbiology: Washington, V. 58, 12, pp. 3834-3836

(29) Slawson, R.M., Van Dyke, M.I., Lee, H. and Trevors, J. T. (1992) Germanium and Silver resistance, accumulation and toxicity in microorganisms. Article found in Plasmid. Academic Press, Inc., San Diego, V. 27, 1, pp. 73-79

(30) Thurman, R. B., and Gerba, C. P. (1989). The molecular mechanisms of copper and silver ion Disinfection of bacteria and viruses. CRC Critical Reviews in Environmental Control, V. 18, 4, p. 295

(31) Ibid., p. 299

(32) Ibid., p. 300

(33) Ibid., p. 301

(34) Ibid., p. 302

(35) Hussain, Saber; Anner, Rolf M.; & anner, Beatrice M.; Cystine protects Na,K-ATPase and isolated human lymphocytes from silver toxicity, Biochemical and Biophysical Research Communications, Vol. 189, No. 3, Dec. 30, 1992, pp. 1444-1449

(36) H.E.L.P.ful NEWS, 12.1.93, Vol. 9, Number 12, pp. 1-3

(37) Duhamel, B. G. M.D.,"Electric Metallic Colloids and their Therapeutical Applications", Lancet, Jan 13, 1912

(38) MacLeod, Alex O. E., "Electric Metallic Colloids and their Therapeutical Applications", Lancet, Feb. 3, 1912

(39) Castle, James, M.D., "Some Recent Observations on Sprue", British Medical Journal, Nov. 15, 1912

(40) Simpson, W. J. M.D., "Experiments on the Germicidal Action of Colloidal Silver", Lancet, Dec. 12, 1914

(41) Marshall, C. R. M.D., and Killoh, G. B. M.D., "The Bactericidal Action of Collosols of Silver and Mercury", British Medical Journal, Jan 16, 1915

(42) Roe, Legge A., "Collosol Argentum and its Ophthalmic uses", British Medical Journal, Jan 16, 1915

(43) Sanderson-Wells, T. H., M.D., "A Case of Puerperal Septicaemia Successfully Treated with Intravenous Injections of Collosol Argentum", Lancet, Feb. 16, 1916

(44) Brown, G. Van Amber, M.D., "Colloidal Silver in Sepsis", Journal of the American Association of Obstetricians and Gynecologists, Jan , 1916

(45) Demant, P., Journal of the American Medical Association, "Blocking the Reticulo-endothelial system and Glycemia", p. 916, 87 (23) Dec. 4, 1926

(46) Shouse, Samuel S., M.D., and Whipple, George H., M.D., "Effects of the Intravenous Injection of Colloidal Silver upon the Hematopoetic System in Dogs", Journal of Experimental Medicine, 53, p. 413-419, 1931

(47) Westhafen, M., Schafer, H., "Generalized Argyrosis in man: Neurological, Ultrastructural and X-ray microanalytical findings", Archives of Otorhinolaryngology, 1986; 232; 260-264

(48) Doull, J. et. al., Cosaret and Doull's Toxicology, The Basic Science of Poisons, Third Edition, 1986, p. 625

(49) Greene, R.M., Su, WP Daniel, "Argyria", American Family Physician, 1987; 36; 151-154

(50) Colloidal Silver Proteins Marketed as Health Supplements, Journal of the American Medical Association, JAMA October 18, 1995 — Vol. 274, No. 15

(51) Materia Medica with Repertory by William Boericke, M.D., Sett Dey & Co., Calcutta, 1976

(52) Physical Therapy Procedures: Selected Techniques, Downer, Ann, B.A., M.A., L.P.T., Charles C Thomas Publisher, 1977

(53) A Manual of Electrotherapy, Schriber, William J., M.A., M.D., Lea & Febiger, 1978

(54) Chiropractic Physiological Therapeutics, Johnson, A.C., D.C., 1977

(55) Handbook of Physical Medicine and Rehabilitation, Krusen, Frank H., M.D., Kottke, Frederic J., M.D., pH.D., Ellwood, Paul M. Jr., M.D., W.B. Saunders Company, 1971

(56) The Pharmacological Basis of Therapeutics, Gillman, , A., Goodman, L.S., 5th ed. New York,: Macmillan, 1975:930-1

(57) The Effect of Electrically Generated Silver Ions on Human Cells, Robert O. Becker, M.D.,Proceedings of the First International Conference on Gold and Silver in Medicine, pg 227-243, The Gold and Silver Institutes, Suite 101, 1026 16th St., N.W., Washington, D.C. 20036

(58) Interaction of Metal Ions and Biological Systems, with special reference to Silver and Gold, Eichhorn, Gunter, et. al., Proceedings of the First International Conference on Gold and Silver in Medicine, pg 3-22, The Gold and Silver Institutes, Suite 101, 1026 16th St., N.W., Washington, D.C. 20036

(59) Silver Anode Inhibition of Bacteria, Spardo, J.A., Proceedings of the First International Conference on Gold and Silver in Medicine, pg 245-260, The Gold and Silver Institutes, Suite 101, 1026 16th St., N.W., Washington, D.C. 20036

(60) Clinical Application of Electrical Silver Iontophoresis, Flick, A.B., Proceedings of the First International Conference on Gold and Silver in Medicine, pg 273-276, The Gold and Silver Institutes, Suite 101, 1026 16th St., N.W., Washington, D.C. 20036

(61) The Biocompatibility of Silver, Williams, D.F., Proceedings of the First International Conference on Gold and Silver in Medicine, pg 261-272, The Gold and Silver Institutes, Suite 101, 1026 16th St., N.W., Washington, D.C. 20036

(62) A Contribution to the pathology of generalized argyria with a discussion of the fate of silver in the human body, Gettler, A.O., et. al., Am J Pathol 1927;3:631-52

(63) Fung, Man C., & Bowen, Debra L., Journal of Toxicology: Clinical Toxicology, Jan 1996, V34 N1, p119(8)

(64) Federal Register Vol. 61, No. 200 Tuesday, October 15, 1996 Proposed Rules 53685, 21 CFR Part 310 [Docket No.96N-0144] Over-the-Counter Drug Products Containing Colloidal Silver ingredients or Silver Salts

(65) Loftus, John & Aarons, Mark, The Secret War Against tne Jews, St. Martin's Press, 1994, pages 293,294 p.83

(66)Schiff, Michael, The Memory of Water, Thorsons, , 1995, ISBN 0 7225 3262 8

(67) Sheldon, J.H., M.D., The British Medical Journal, Jan 13, 1934, p. 47-58

(68) Bellavite, Paolo, M.D. & Signorini, M.D., HOMEOPATHY: A Frontier In Medical Science, North Atlantic Books, 1995, ISBN 1-55643-211-9

(69) Berg, A.O., Placebos: A Brief Review for Family Physicians, J. Fam. Pract., 1977, July; 5(1):97-100

(70) Farber, Paul M., N.D., D.C., PhD., The Micro Silver Bullet, 1995, ISBN 1887742-00-X

(71) Daryl Tichy Updates, A newsletter published by Daryl Tichy,349 North 250 East, Orem, Utah 84057, Several issues from 1994-1996

(72) Silver Colloids - Do They Work? by Ronald J. Gibbs, ISBN: 0967699207, 1999 http://www.amazon.com/Silver-Colloids-Do-They-Work/dp/0967699207

(73) Beyond Antibiotics : Boost Your Immunity and Avoid Antibiotics by Michael A. Schmidt, Lendon H. Smith (Contributor), Keith W. Sehnert Contributor), North Atlantic Books, 1994, ISBN: 1556431805

(74) Colloidal Silver. Where does it go when you drink it? How long does it stay there?, By Roger Altman, Eng. Sc. D. , 1999, rogaltman@aol.com
http://www.silvermedicine.org/AltmanStudy.pdf

(75) Becker, Robert O., Effects of Electrically Generated Silver Ions on Human Cells and Wound Healing, Electro- and Magnetobiology, 19(1), 1-19, 2000

(76) Bach A.,Boher H., Motsch J., Martin E., Geiss H.K., Sonntag H.G., Prevention of bacterial colonization of intravenous catheters by antiseptic impregnation of polyurethane polymers J of Antimicrob Chem. ,33:969-978, 1994

(77) Becker R.O., Spadaro J.A. ,Treatment of Orthopedic Infections with Electrically Generated Silver Ions J. Bone Jt. Surgery 60-A:871,1978

(78) Chu C.C., Tsai W.C., Yao J.Y. ,Chiu S.S., Newly made antibacterial braided nylon sutures. 1. In vitro qualitative and in vivo preliminary biocompatibility studyJ. Biomed. Material Res., 21:1281, 1987

(79) Chu C.S., McManus A.T., Mason A.D., Okerberg C.V., Pruitt B.A. Multiple Graft Harvestings from Deep Partial-thickness Scald Wounds Healed under the Influence of Weak Direct Current Journal of Trauma, 30:1044, 1990

(80) Chu C.S., McManus A.T., Matylevich N., Mason A.D., Pruitt B.A., Direct Current Reduces Wound Edema After Full Thickness Burn Injury in Rats Journal of Trauma, Injury, Infection & Critical Care, 400 (5):738, 1990

(81) Chu C.S., McManus A.T.,Okerberg C.V.,Mason A.D., Pruitt B.A. Weak Direct Current Accelerates Split-thickness Graft Healing on Tangentially Excised Second-degree Burns J of Burn Care Rehab, 12:285-293, 1991

(82) Chu C.S., McManus A.T. Pruitt B.A., Mason A.D., Theraputic Effects of Silver Nylon Dressings with Weak Direct Current on Pseudomonas aeruginosa-Infected Burn Wounds The Journal of Trauma,28(10):1488-1492, 1988

(83) Clement J.L., Jarrett P.S., Antibacterial Silver Metal Based Drugs 1(56):467-482, 1994

(84) Deitch E.A., Malaleonok A.A., Albright J.A., Electric Augmentation of the Anti-Bacterial Activity of Silver-Nylon, 3rd Annual BRAGS, 10/2-5/1983

(85) Deitch E.A., Marino A.A., Gillespie T.E., Albright J.A., Silver-Nylon: A New Antimicrobial Agent, Antimicrobial Agents Chemother., 23:356, 1983

(86) Maki D.G., Garman J.K., Shapiro J.M., Ringer M.,Helgerson R.B., An Attachable Silver-Impregnated Cuff for Prevention of Infection with Central Venous Catheters: A Prospective Randomized Multicenter Trial Attachable Silver, Am J of Med, 85:307-314, 1988

(87) Maki D.G., Stolz S.M., Wheeler A., Mermel L.A., Prevention of Central Venous Catheter-Related Blookstream Infection by Use of an Antiseptic-Impregnated Catheter, Am College of Physicians, 127(4):257-266, 5 Aug 1997

(88) Marino A.A.,Deitch E.A., Albright J.A., Electric Silver Antisepsis, IEEE Trans. Biomed. Eng.BME, 32:336, 1985

(89) Marino A.A., Deitch E.A., Malakanok V., Albright J.A., Specian R.D., Electrical Augmentation of the Antimicrobial Activity of Silver-Nylon Fabrics, J. Biol. Phys., 12:93, 1984

(90) Marino A.A., Malakonok V., Albright J.A., Deitch E.A., Specian R.D., Electrochemical properties of silver-nylon fabrics, J. of Electrochem Soc.,132:68,1985

(91) Nand S., Sengar G.K., Nand S., Jain V.K., Gupta T.D., Dual Use of Silver for A Management of Chronic Bone Infections and Infected Non- Unions, J. Indian Medical Assoc, 84:134-136, 1996

(92) Sheridan R., Doherty P.J. Gilchrist T., Healy D., The effect of antibacterial agents on the behariour of Cultured Mammalian Fibroblasts., J. of Materials Science, 6:853-856, 1995

(93) Spadaro J.A., Kramer S.J., Webster D.A., Antibacterial demineralized bone matrix using silver, 28th Annual ORS- , N. Orleans, LA, Jan 19-21,1982

(94) Spadaro J.A., Webster D.A., Chapin S.E., Yuan H.A., Murray D.G., Becker R.O., Silver-PMMA Antibacterial bone cement , 24th Annual

(95) Spadaro J.A., Webster D.A., Becker R.O., Silver Polymethyl methacrylate antibacterial bone cement Clinical Orthop, 143:266, 1979

(96) Spadaro J.A., Webster D.A., Kovach D.A., Chase S.E., Antibacterial Fixation Pins wth Silver: Animal Models, Trans Orthop Res Soc, 9:335, 1984

(97) Tsai W.C., Chu C.C., Chin S.S., Yao J.Y., In Vitro quantitative study of newly made antibacterial braided nylon sutures, Surg. Gynecol. Obstet., 165:207, 1987

(98) Webster D.A., Spadaro J.A., Kramer S., Becker R.O., Silver Anode treatment of chronic osteomyelitis, Clin Orthop, 1961:105, 1981

(99) Williams D.F., The Biocompatibility of Silver, 1st Int'l Conf Gold & Silver, Bethesda, MD, May 13-14,

(100) Williams R.L., Doherty P.J., Vince D.G., Grashoff G. J., Williams D.F., The Biocompability of Silver, Critical Reviews in Biocompatibility, 5:221, 1989

(101) http://www.incore.com/india/commun.ayurveda.html#metal

(102) http://www.silvermedicine.org/argyria.html - Accessed On 9/25/2008

(103) Silver (CASRN 7440-22-4) EPA Integrated Risk Management System - http://www.epa.gov/iris/subst/0099.htm - Accessed on 9/25/2008

(104) http://www.eytonsearth.org/forum/about7.html

(105) http://www.natural-immunogenics.com/pdf/Rentz_-_Jl_Nutritional_&_Environemntal_Medicine_-_Jun_2003.pdf

(106) Jun Tian, Dr. , Kenneth K. Y. Wong, Dr.[1][*], Chi-Ming Ho, Dr. , Chun-Nam Lok, Dr., Wing-Yiu Yu, Dr., Chi-Ming Che, Prof. , Jen-Fu Chiu, Prof.[3], Paul K. H. Tam, Prof., Topical Delivery of Silver Nanoparticles Promotes Wound Healing, Department of Surgery, Li Ka Shing Faculty of Medicine, University of Hong Kong, Queen Mary Hospital, Hong Kong SAR, China,   Department of Chemistry, University of Hong Kong, Hong Kong SAR, China Department of Anatomy, Li Ka Shing Faculty of Medicine, University of Hong Kong, Hong Kong SAR, China

(107) Becker, Robert O., Induced Dedifferentialtion: A possible alternative to embryonic stem cell transplants, Neurorehabilitation 17 (2002) 23-34

(108) Dean W, Mitchell M, Whizar Lugo V, South J. Reduction of Viral Load in AIDS Patients with Intravenous Mild Silver Protein-- Three Case Reports. Clinical Practice of Alternative Medicine. Spring, 2001.

(109) R. P. Andres et al., "Research Opportunities on Cluster and Cluster-Assembled Materials", J. Mater. Res. Vol. 4, No 3, 1989, p. 704.

(110) The Pharmacological Basis of Therapeutics, Fifth Edition, by Louis S. Goodman and Alfred Gilman (editors), published by MacMillan Publishing Company, NY, 1975

(111) I. B. Romans, Disinfection, Sterlization and Preservation, C. A. Lawrence and S. S. Bloek (editors), Lea and Fibiger (1968)

(112) "The Oligodynamic Effect of Silver" by A. Goetz, R. L. Tracy and F. S. Harris, Jr. in Silver in Industry, Lawrence Addicks (editor), published by Reinhold Publishing Corporation, 1940.

(113) **2072 Federal Register** / Vol. 74, No. 9 / Wednesday, January 14, 2009 / Notices

(114) http://www.regulations.gov/fdmspublic/component/main?main=SubmitComment&o=090000648081edc9 Accessed on 3/5/2009

(115) http://www.healthiertalk.com/battle-save-colloidal-silver-regulation-epa-0236 Accessed on 3/5/2009

(116) Russell, A.D., et al. 1994. Antimicrobial activity and action of silver. Progress in Medicinal Chemistry, 31, 351-370

(117) Antelman, Marvin S. 1994. Silver (II, III) disinfectants. Soap/Cosmetics/Specialties. March: 52-59.

(118) Feng, Q.L., et al. 2000. A mechanistic study of the antibacterial effect of silver ions on Escherichia coli and Staphylococcus Aureus. Journal of Biomedical Materials Research, 52, 662-668.

(119) Chambers, Cecil W., Proctor, Charles M., and Kabler, Paul W. 1962. Bactericidal effect of low concentrations of silver. Journal of the American Water Works Association, 208-216.

(120) Miller, Lawrence P., and McCallan, S.E.A. 1957. Toxic action of metal ions to fungus spores. Agricultural and Food Chemistry, 5(2), 116-122.

(121) Carr, Howard S., Wlodkowski, Theodore J., and Rosenkranz, Herbert S. 1973. Silver sulfadiazine: in vitro antibacterial activity. *Antimicrobial Agents and Chemotherapy*, 4(5), 585-587.

(122) Rendin, Larry J, Gamba, Carl L., and Johnson, Walllace M. 1958. Colloidal oxide of silver in the treatment of peptic ulcer. *Pennsylvania Medical Journal*. 61: 612-614.

(123) Motohashi, Shinzo. 1922. Fixed-tissue phagocytosis. Journal of Medical Research. 43: 419-434.

(124) Samuni A, et al. On the Cytotoxicity of Vitamin C and metal ions. *Eur J Biochem*. 1983;99:562.

(125) Jansson G. Harms-Ringdahl M. Stimulating effects of mercuric- and silver ions on the superoxide anion in human polymorphonuclear leukocytes. *Free Radic Res Commun*, 1993;18(2):87-98.

(126) Horsmanheimo, M. Lack of proliferation of circulating white blood cells in patients with syphilis before and after a Jarisch-Herxheimer Reaction. *Br J Vener Dis*. 1978 Aug;54:225-8.

(127) Loveday C, Bingham JS. Changes in circulating immune complexes during the Jarisch Herxheimer Reaction in secondary Syphilis. *Eur J Clin Microbiol Infect Dis*. 1993 Mar;12:185-91.

(128) Rikimaru T, et al. Three cases of localized pleural Tuberculosis which looked exacerbated during antituberculous chemotherapy. *Kekkaku*. 1991 Feb;66:101-7.

(129) Karachunskii MA. Exacerbation of pulmonary Tuberculosis during chemotherapy. *Probl Tuberk*, 1996;23-5.

(130) Lawrence C, et al. Seronegative chronic relapsing Neuroborreliosis. *Eur Neurol*, 1995;35:113-7.

(131) Berg D, Berg LH, Couvaras J. Is CFS/FM due to an undefined hypercoagulable state brought on by immune activation of coagulation? Does adding anticoagulant therapy improve CFS/FM patient symptoms? *AACFS Proceedings*: Cambridge, MA. 1998 Oct 10-12;62.

(132) Eric Gordon, MD and Kent Holtorf, MD, A Promising Cure for URTI Pandemics, Including H5N1 and SARS: Has the Final Solution to the Coming Plagues Been Discovered? (Part II) , April 2006 http://www.gordonresearch.com/Presentations/GRI_mar07/articles/promising_cure.html Accessed on March 18, 2009

(133) Lok CN, Ho CM, Chen R, He QY, Yu WY, Sun H, Tam PK, Chiu JF, Che CM., Silver nanoparticles: partial oxidation and antibacterial activities, J Biol Inorg Chem, 2007 May;12(4):527-34. Epub 2007 Feb

(134) Kim JS, Kuk E, Yu KN, Kim JH, Park SJ, Lee HJ, Kim SH, Park YK, Park YH, Hwang CY, Kim YK, Lee YS, Jeong DH, Cho MH., Abtimicrobial effects of silver nanoparticles, Nanomedicine, 2007 Mar;3(1):95-101.

(135) Bacterial Silver resistance: molecular biology and uses and misuses of silver compounds, FEMS Microbiol Rev., 2003 Jun;27(2-3):341-53

(136) Li L, Zhu YJ, High chemical reactivity of silver nanoparticles toward hydrochloric, J Colloid Interface Sci, 2006 Nov 15;303(2):415-8. Epub 2006 Jul 27

9 781884 979088